Scars

Edited by Anca Chiriac

Published in London, United Kingdom

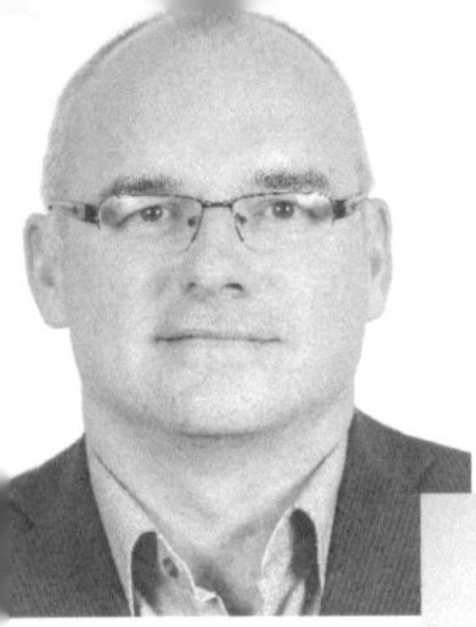

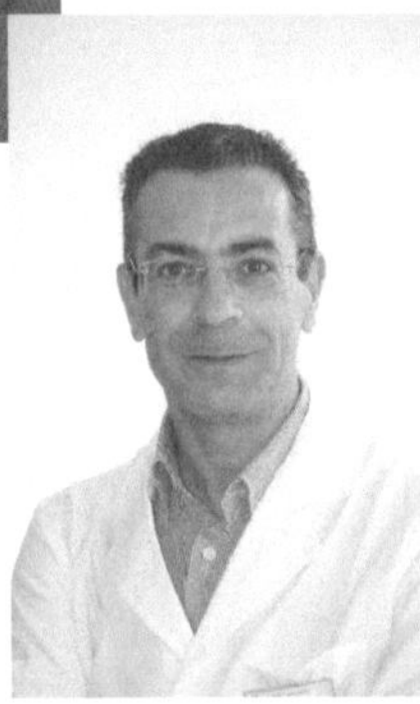

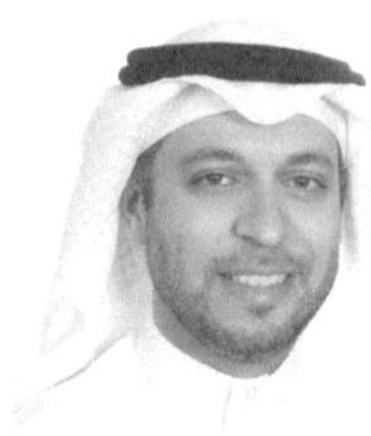

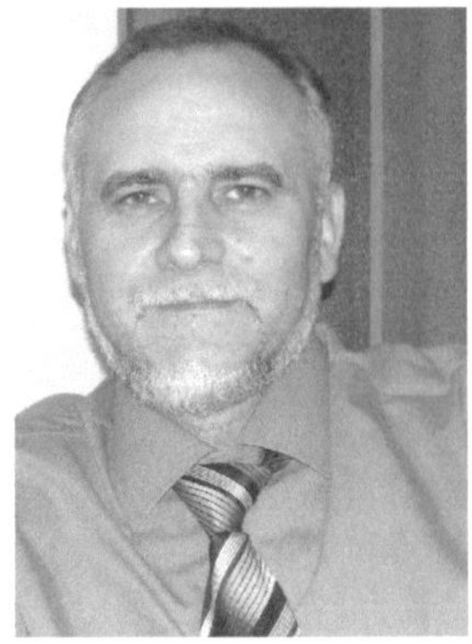

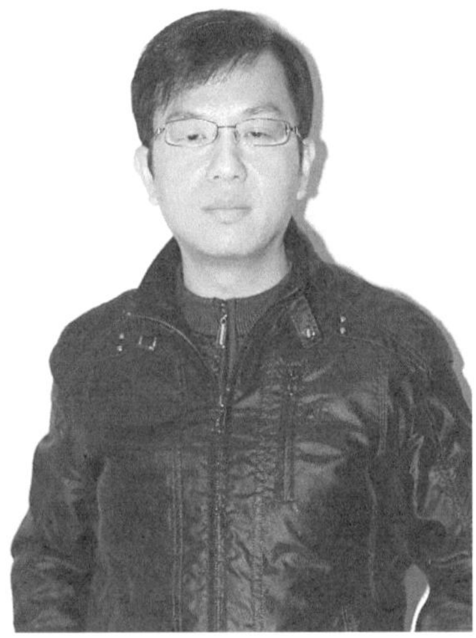

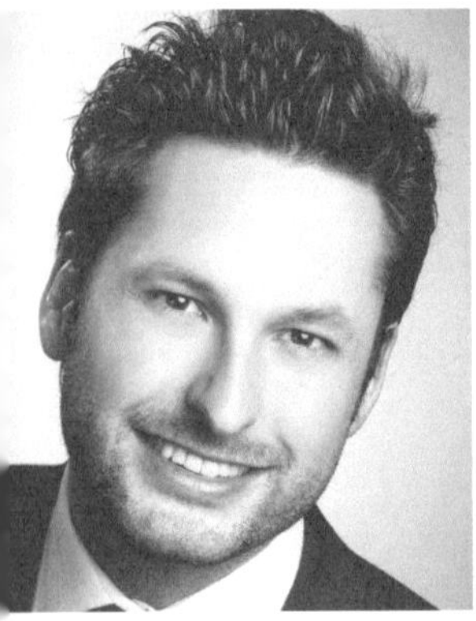

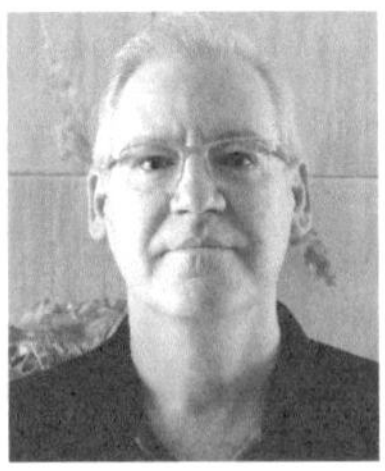

IntechOpen

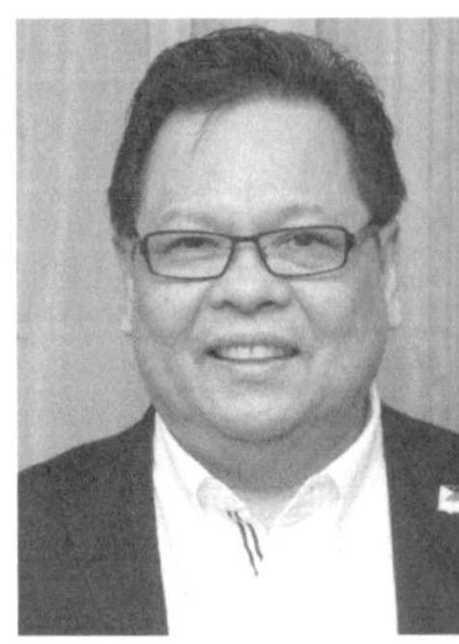

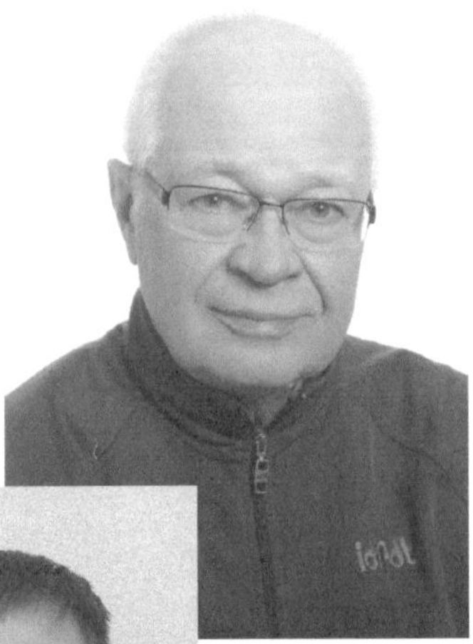

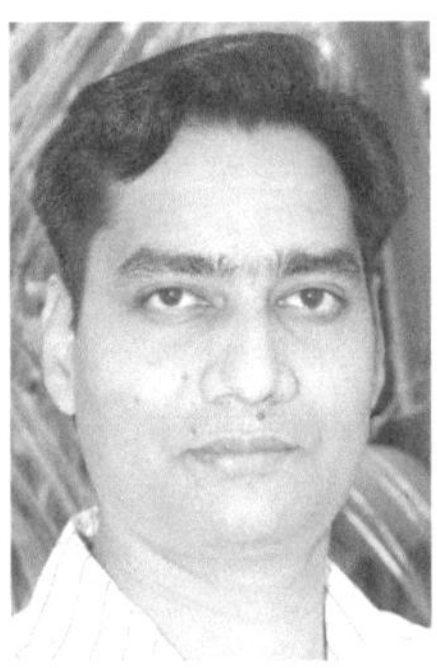

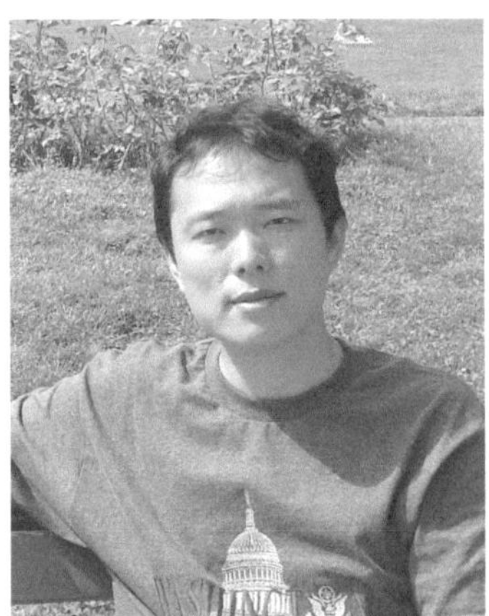

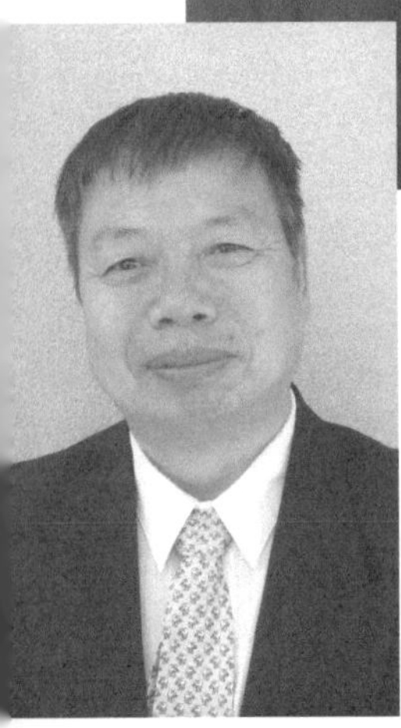

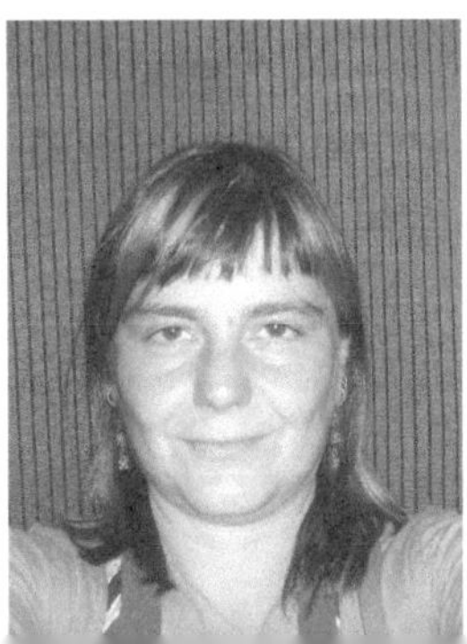

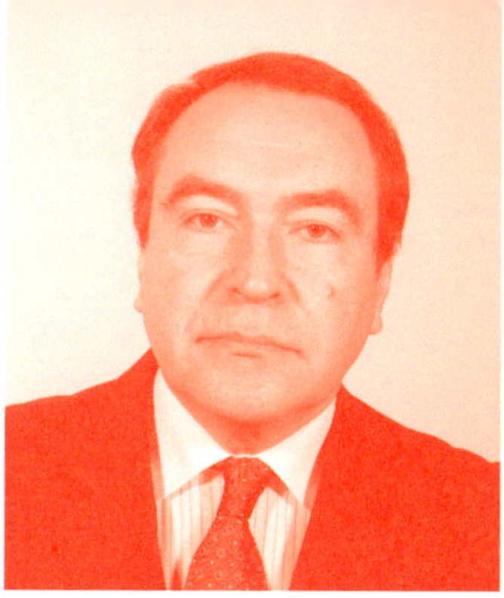

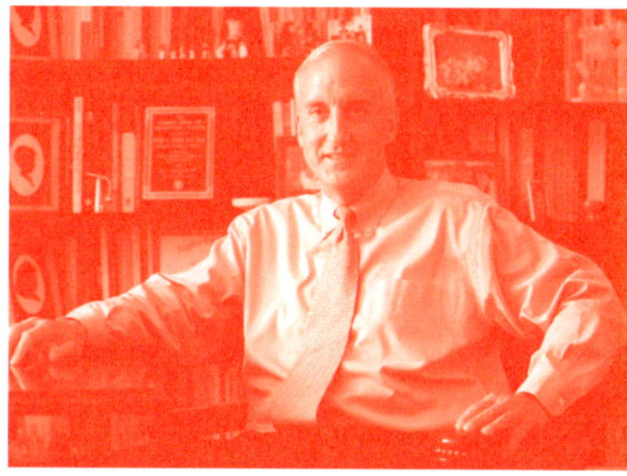

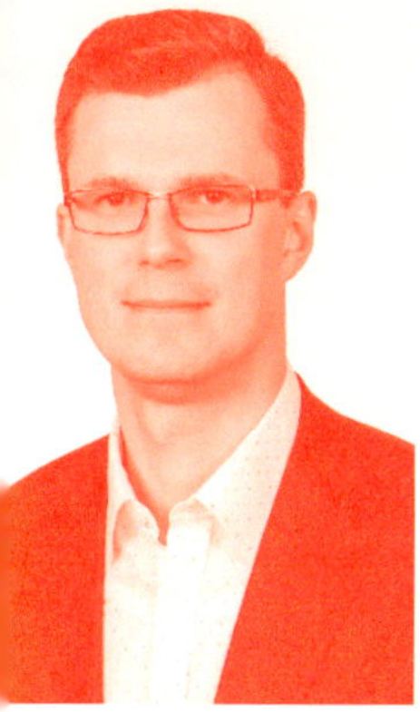

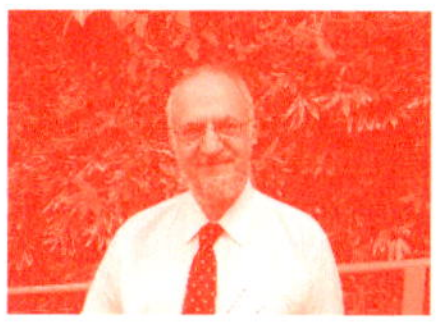

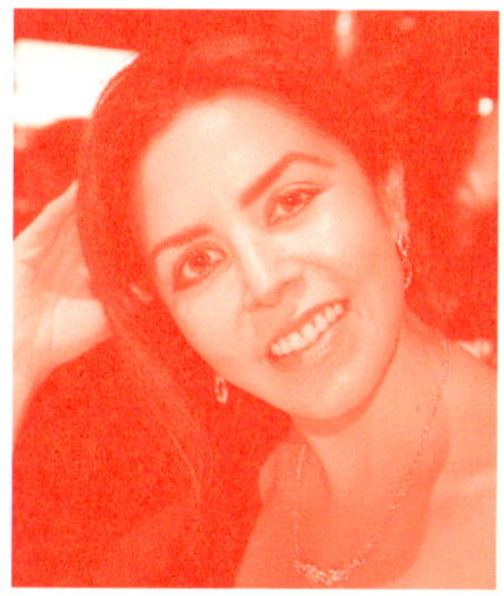

Supporting open minds since 2005

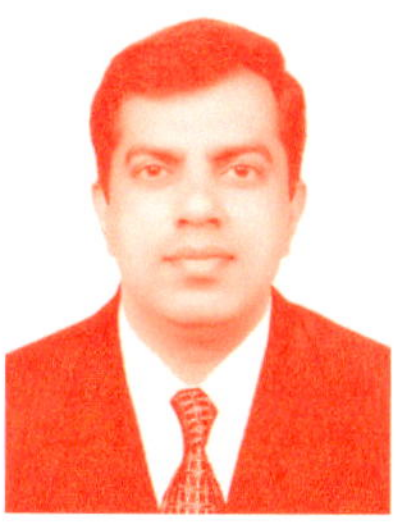

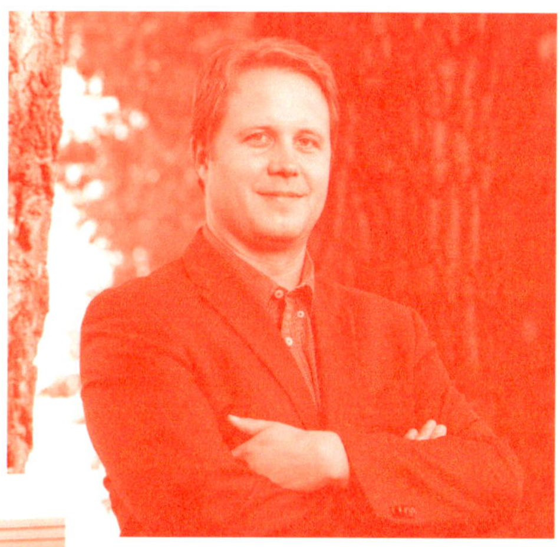

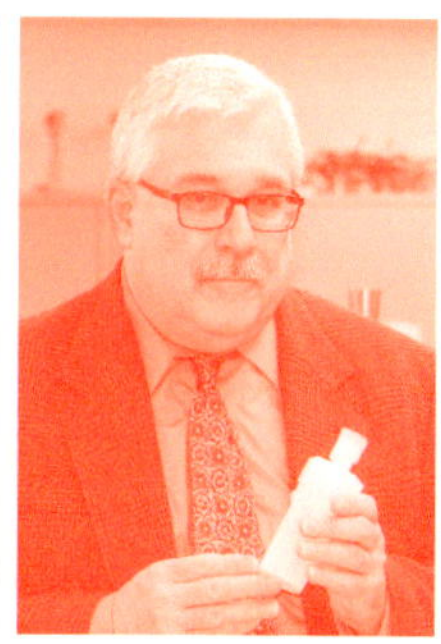

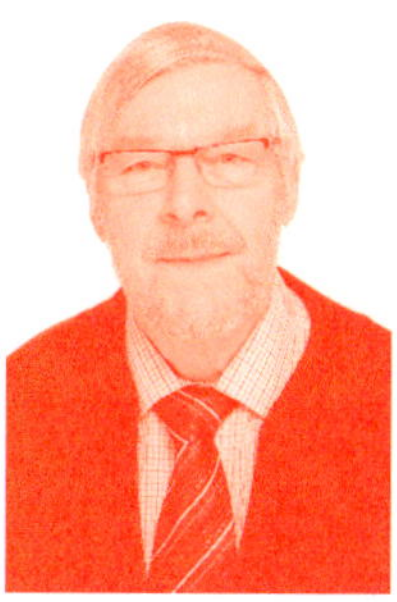

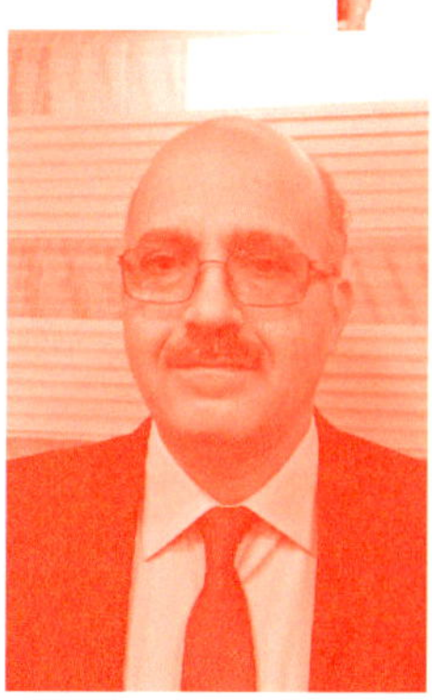

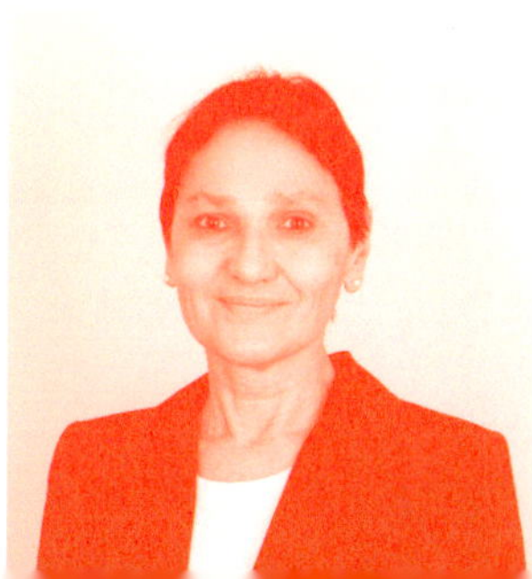

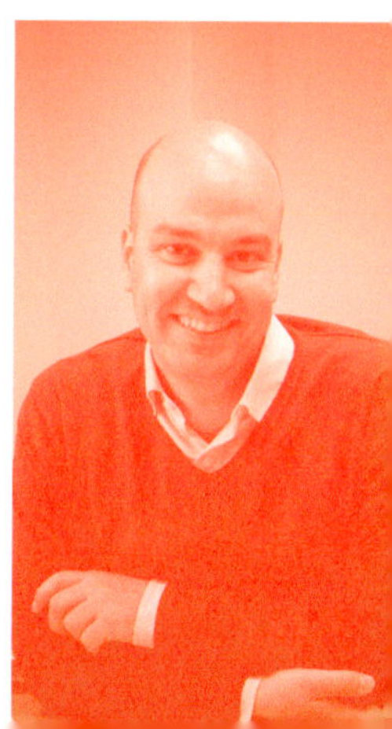

Scars
http://dx.doi.org/10.5772/intechopen.73982
Edited by Anca Chiriac

Contributors
Andrei Plotski, Rei Ogawa, Gustavo Prezzavento, Iyadh Ghorbel, Slim Moalla, Amal Abid, Amir Karra, Khalil Ennouri, Lindsay Damkat-Thomas, John E. Greenwood, Anca Chiriac

First published in London, United Kingdom, 2019 by IntechOpen
IntechOpen is the global imprint of INTECHOPEN LIMITED, registered in England and Wales, registration number: 11086078, The Shard, 25th floor, 32 London Bridge Street
London, SE19SG - United Kingdom
Printed in Croatia

British Library Cataloguing-in-Publication Data
A catalogue record for this book is available from the British Library

Additional hard and PDF copies can be obtained from orders@intechopen.com

Scars
Edited by Anca Chiriac
p. cm.
Print ISBN 978-1-83880-934-8
Online ISBN 978-1-83881-892-0
eBook (PDF) ISBN 978-1-83881-893-7

Meet the editor

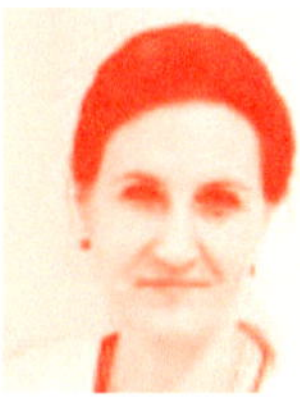

Anca Chiriac is Full Professor of Dermatology and Venereology at Apollonia University, a clinical dermatologist at Nicolina Medical Center and "Saint Mary" Emergency Hospital for Children, and a researcher at "P. Poni" Institute of Macromolecular Chemistry, Iasi, Romanian Academy. She graduated in 1991 at "Grigore T. Popa" University of Medicine and Pharmacy, Iasi, and received her PhD in Medicine in 2005 at "C. Davila" University of Medicine and Pharmacy, Bucharest, Romania.
She has authored more than 250 articles, chapters, and books and has been involved in many international research projects.

Contents

Preface

"Scarring is a natural part of the healing process" as defined by Wikipedia (https://en.wikipedia.org/wiki/Scar) and underlines the coexistence of two processes: injury and healing.

Thus, a scar is a mark of life, beyond a simple medical problem. Its impact on us as human beings is greater than one can imagine.

Scars are present even in art collections, for example the painting *SCAR* by German artist J. Coblenz. Scarring is also well symbolized in ancient Chinese art. Music uses the idea of scar with metaphoric symbols in the lyrics of different songs, for example "Scar Tissue" by the Red Hot Chili Peppers has wonderful and powerful words. Movies have caught the attention of scar too with the film *SCAR* released in 2007 or, more recently, *Sharp Objects* from 2018.

Scars are parts of our lives and extensively we can admit that almost everyone has one.

Skin scarring is an important medical problem, and is a main concern for patients, physicians, and researchers who deal with cutaneous injury and repair. Deciphering the process of scarring and finding new methods to treat "ugly" scars remain tenacious aims for many researchers from around the world.

Anca Chiriac
Professor,
Nicolina Medical Center,
Department of Dermatology,
Iasi, Romania Apollonia University,
Iasi, Romania

Petru Poni Institute of Macromolecular Chemistry,
Iasi, Romanian Academy

"Saint Mary" Emergency Children's Hospital,
Iasi, Romania

Section 1

Scars

Chapter 1

Introductory Chapter: Scars

Anca Chiriac

1. Overview

Scar is the result of the process of wound healing that, finally, modifies the normal skin morphology. Wound healing process is very complex and incomplete elucidated, but it is based on four major processes: coagulation, inflammation, proliferation, and remodeling [1].

Dermal injury, especially reticular dermis damage, induces permanent scars [2].

In daily practice one can admit that every person can have their particular scarring process, provoking an important negative impact on quality of life, due to cosmetic, physical, physiological, and, sometimes, disfiguring effects.

If the inflammatory process is too intense, it can initiate abnormal fibroblast proliferation and excessive collagen, resulting keloids or hypertrophic scars. If collagen degradation is more intense than collagen synthesis, the result is an atrophic scar [3]. Keloid is different from hypertrophic by its margins which extend beyond the limits of the initial wound, whatever the type.

Different types of scars can develop after variable type of skin wounds, caused by a large variety of factors, ranging from simple trauma to surgery, from therapeutic methods (laser) to inflammatory skin disorders (acne). "Spontaneous" keloids can be diagnosed, in the absence of any sign of skin injury, especially in young adults, more often located on the upper back.

On the other hand, the type of skin scar is influenced by many factors: genetic predisposition, skin structure, age and gender, race, comorbidities, or/and systemic or local treatment corroborated with type, depth, and location of skin injury [4]. Anatomical area can influence the type of scarring; thorax and superior limbs are most likely to develop hypertrophic and keloid scars, while this type of scarring is never seen on the eyelids [5].

The cause of skin injury plays an important role in pathological scarring. Burns of different degrees are followed by hypertrophic scars, especially if the deep dermis is affected, in predisposed individuals and in the presence of skin infection [6]. Keloids have been reported after non-intense but chronic trauma, for example, ear piercing [6]. Scarring in acne, in adolescents, is atrophic type and difficult to manage.

Burns raise difficulties in therapy not only in acute phase but also when pathological scarring occurred. Hypertrophic scars develop 1–2 months after burns, while keloids can be observed much later, even years.

Scars can be asymptomatic or accompanied by pruritus or pain, but major concern is esthetic anxiety.

Scars are treated by an interdisciplinary team, plastic surgeon, dermatologist, family care physician, and specialized nurse. Variable guidelines are available, but treatment of a pathological scar remains, even nowadays a challenge.

Within the pages of each chapter of the book *Scar*, new insights in definition, etiology, pathogenic mechanism, and therapeutic methods are described. The book

IntechOpen

is a guideline for medical care providers who treat patients with scars but also can open new doors for understanding and treating pathological scarring.

The introductory chapter presents clinical images of skin scars (**Figures 1–7**), in order to show the huge impact on quality of life of patients and the difficulties and limitations of physicians treating such lesions.

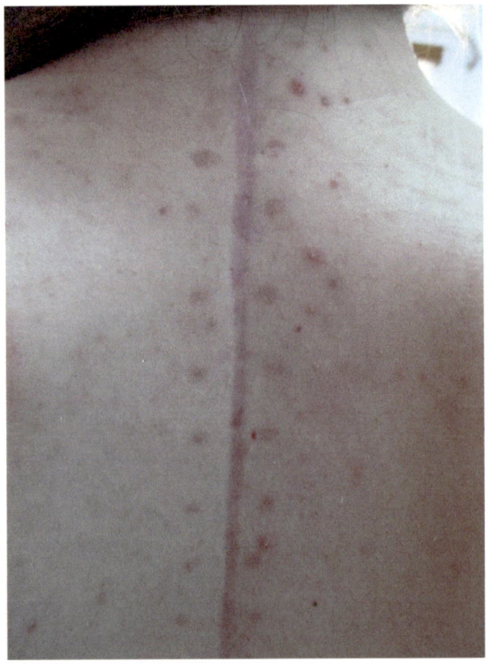

Figure 1.
Recent postsurgery scar.

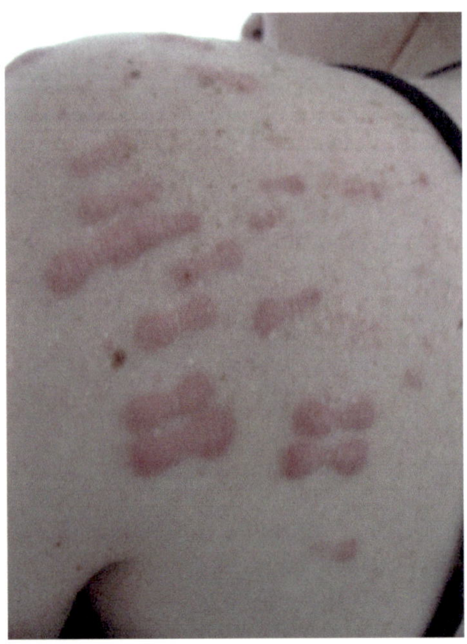

Figure 2.
"Spontaneous" keloids.

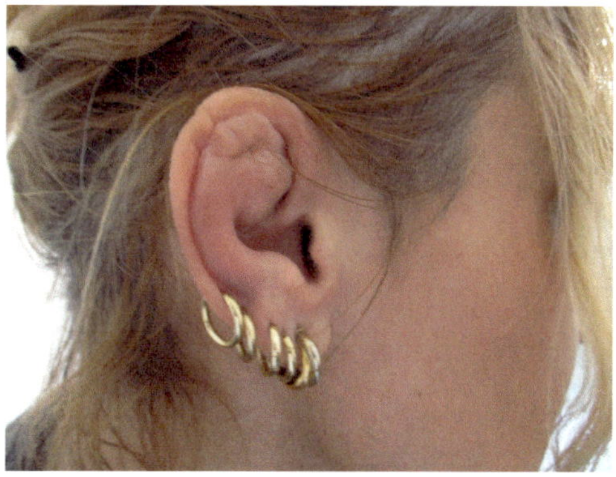

Figure 3.
Keloids after ear piercing.

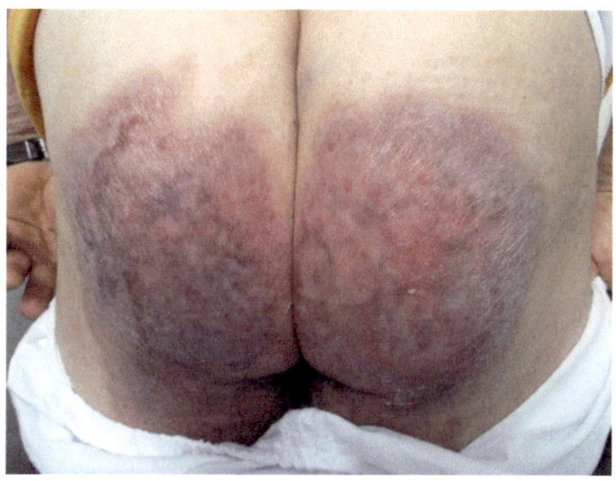

Figure 4.
Atrophic scar after electrical burn.

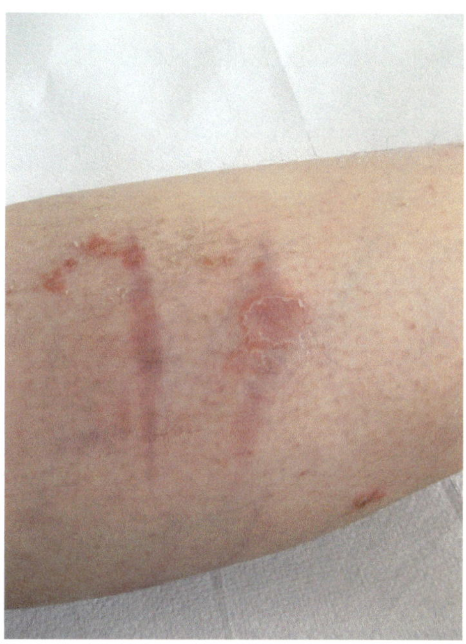

Figure 5.
Striae induced by prolonged use of topical potent steroids.

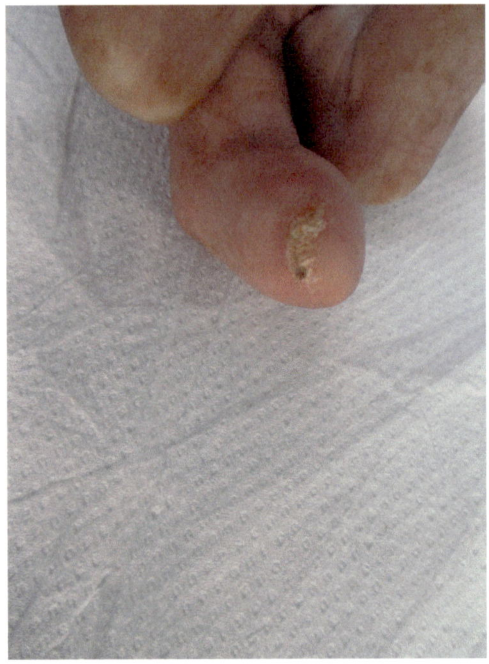

Figure 6.
Squamous cell carcinoma arising within the margins of an ancient caustic burn.

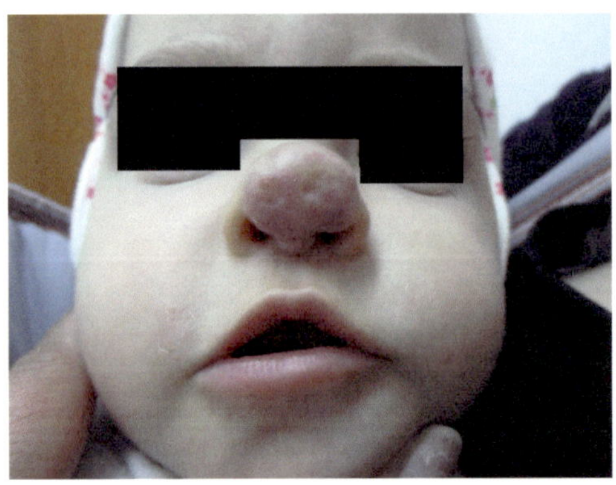

Figure 7.
Atrophic scar after bleomycin injected for vascular anomaly.

Author details

Anca Chiriac[1,2,3,4*]

1 Nicolina Medical Center, Department of Dermatology, Iasi-Romania

2 Apollonia University, Iasi-Romania

3 "P.Poni" Institute of Macromolecular Chemistry, Iasi, Romanian Academy

4 "Saint Mary" Emergency Children Hospital Iasi, Romania

*Address all correspondence to: ancachiriac@yahoo.com

References

[1] Ogawa R. Surgery for scar revision and reduction: From primary closure to flap surgery. Burns & Trauma. 2019;7:7

[2] Niessen FB, Spauwen PH, Schalkwijk J, Kon M. On the nature of hypertrophic scars and keloids: A review. Plastic and Reconstructive Surgery. 1999;**104**(5):1435-1458

[3] Wolfram D, Tzankov A, Pülzl P, Piza-Katzer H. Hypertrophic scars and keloids: A review of their pathophysiology, risk factors, and therapeutic management. Dermatologic Surgery. 2009;**35**(2):171-181

[4] Khatri KA, Mahoney DL, McCartney MJ. Laser scar revision: A review. Journal of Cosmetic and Laser Therapy. 2011;**13**(2):54-62

[5] Rodrigues M, Kosaric N, Bonham CA, Gurtner GC. Wound healing: A cellular perspective. Physiological Reviews. 2019;**99**(1):665-706

[6] Schmieder SJ, Ferrer-Bruker SJ. Hypertrophic Scarring. [Updated 2019 Feb 18]. In: StatPearls [Internet]. Treasure Island (FL): StatPearls Publishing; Jan 2019. Available from: https://www.ncbi.nlm.nih.gov/books/NBK470176

Section 2

Burn Scars

Chapter 2

Scarring After Burn Injury

Lindsay Damkat-Thomas and John Edward Greenwood

Abstract

Burn injury is a trauma that has variable scarring outcomes dependent on both the size and the depth of the burn. This chapter will discuss the pathophysiology of wound healing by both primary and secondary intention and its applicability to burn wounds. The importance of accurate assessment of burn depth and its impact on the primary treatment and subsequent scar outcome will be explored. Special anatomic areas such as the face, hands and neck will be highlighted. Skin grafting and skin substitutes as treatment options will be reviewed. Improvements in burn care have enabled people to survive larger burns that may once have proved fatal. The emphasis of treatment, once healing has been achieved, is now focused upon rehabilitation and scar management. Scar management strategies including pressure garments and silicone therapy are highlighted along with secondary scar revision strategies.

Keywords: burn scars, burn surgeon, extensive deep burn injury

1. Introduction

Scarring in the aftermath of burn injury is generally perceived (at least by the media and the general public) to be universally both horribly disfiguring and permanently disabling [1]. In reality, the majority of the outcomes that we achieve as burn surgeons are both functionally and aesthetically excellent. Poor outcomes do occur; however these almost exclusively follow the deepest and most extensive burn injuries. The outcome picture is complicated somewhat because certain burn aetiologies are destined to proffer poorer outcomes. One example is the injuries caused by high-voltage-driven electrical current conduction. Such insult is often associated with major limb amputations, which markedly diminish outcome, and this might be expected [2, 3]. However, even when comparing the scarring outcome from an identical aetiology, such as flame burns, the skin injury sustained in a house fire and affecting a high proportion of the total body surface area often generates significantly poorer outcomes than flame injuries from, for example, localised clothing ignition from being too close to a naked flame. This is despite the skin being damaged to the same depth in both scenarios. It could be surmised that the differences in the environment of the burn injury might result in additional injuries (such as smoke inhalation [4]), which will affect treatment course and even survival. However, if all other parameters are negated, extensive burns are associated with poorer scarring outcomes than small burns of the same depth caused by the same agent [5, 6]. The focus of this chapter is to elucidate why this is the case and to suggest strategies to improve scarring outcome, function and appearance in extensive deep burn injury.

2. Wound healing: primary versus secondary healing

Before discussing burn injuries, the essential tenets of the process of wound healing must be understood by the reader in order to appreciate the strategies employed in managing burn injuries [7]. The essential components of wound healing occur in the dermis. This mesodermal derivative is incapable of regenerating molecular structure and undergoes instead a process of repair driven by the simultaneous deposition of (predominantly) Type III collagen by fibroblasts, and small blood vessel angiogenesis, succeeding an inflammatory response secondary to vascular fluid and protein leakage into the interstitium surrounding the wound and the attraction of circulating polymorphonuclear neutrophils, lymphocytes and monocytes [8]. The dermal repair provides sufficient structure for re-epithelialisation from the approximated wound edges. The epidermis is ectodermal in origin, cellular in composition and capable of regeneration.

In *primary wound healing*, where the wound edges are in close proximity, haemostasis is followed by inflammation and cellular wound debridement, and the dermal fibroblasts rapidly produce collagen to bridge the 'narrow' gap and restore resistance of the skin to external forces [9]. The ratio of collagens in the resulting repair (Type I:III = 1:3) is different than in uninjured skin (Type I:III = 3:1). Type III collagen is not cross-linked and thus has a greater volume than Type I collagen, so the scar is raised above the surrounding skin, and the proliferation of angiogenetic vessels gives it a red appearance. As the scar undergoes maturation, the normal collagen ratio is re-established, the scar volume decreases, and the scar becomes flat, or even depressed, and vascular involution sees it change colour, becoming pale, and resulting in the typical final appearance of the incisional scar.

In *secondary intention healing*, there is considerable tissue loss, and the wound edges are very far apart. Delayed wound closure results. A prolonged inflammatory phase overlaps with excessive deposition of collagen and glycosaminoglycans by dermal fibroblasts and circulating stem cells, accompanied by heavy vascular proliferation (granulation tissue formation) [10]. Polymorphonuclear leukocytes are present to phagocytose bacteria. Since edge epithelialisation can extend only about 5 mm across the wound, myofibroblast differentiation occurs, and these cells act to contract the wound edges to reduce the size in the wound bed to facilitate re-epithelialisation. This results in contracture and problematic scarring [11].

3. The importance of the depth of burn injury

In real terms, there are only two burn 'depths' (**Figure 1**). Most of the burn injuries seen for emergency assessment and treatment are, with optimal support and good wound management, superficial enough to heal spontaneously, quickly and with an excellent functional and cosmetic result. These are burns individually classified as epidermal, superficial partial thickness and mid-dermal, even though the treatment priorities for all are the same—the *prevention of infection* (which can deepen the injury) and the *control of pain* (which facilitates dressing changes, compliance with therapy and mobilisation and hastens discharge) [12, 13]. Then there are those burns that are sufficiently deep to undergo prolonged healing by *secondary intention* (granulation tissue formation and wound contraction), often complicated by recurrent episodes of wound infection, resulting in 'pathological' scarring that

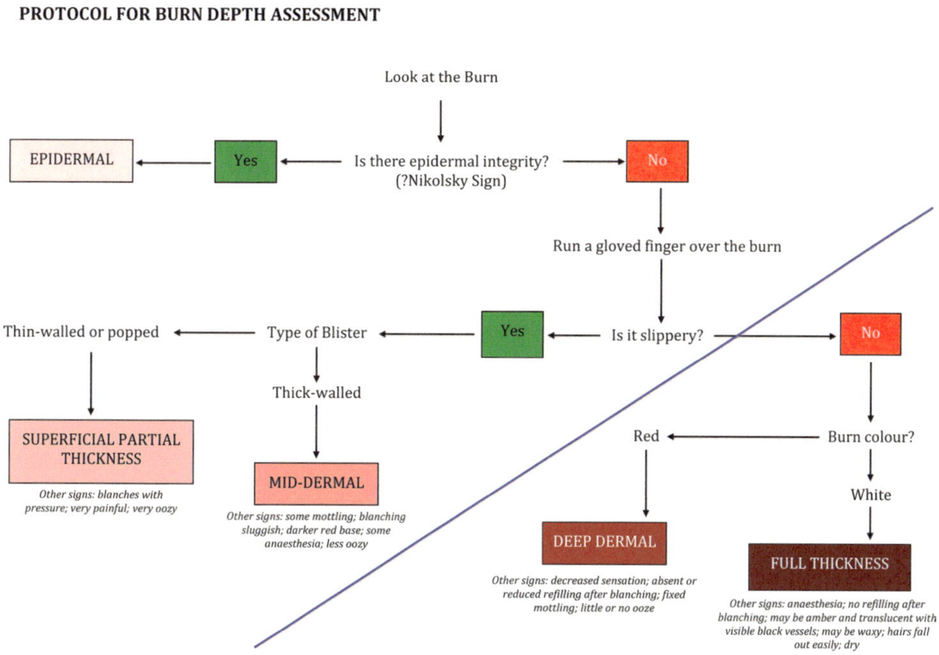

Figure 1.
Flow chart indicating burn depth: the blue diagonal line represents the boundary between those burns with the ability to heal spontaneously (above the line) and those that will require surgical excision and reconstruction to facilitate healing (below the line) [12]. This method must be used within 24–36 h post-injury since burn wound exudation is required for depth determination.

reduces, impairs or abolishes function and is hypertrophic, dysaesthetic and often symptomatic (causing itching and pain). It is this second group that contains those burns described clinically as 'deep dermal' and 'full thickness'. The treatment priority in these burns is to *abort the process of secondary intention healing and replace it, as closely as possible with primary intention healing*.

3.1 Spontaneously healing burns

For the purposes of this chapter, it is enough to understand that those burns in that spontaneously healing group are sufficiently superficial that there is a volume of good viable residual dermal tissue in the burn bed as well as the survival of multiple nests of epidermal stem cells (keratinocyte progenitor cells) located in the invaginated sheathes of the adnexal structures (hair follicles, sweat glands and sebaceous glands) [14, 15]. These cells can differentiate into keratinocytes, proliferate and migrate across the viable dermis to effect rapid re-epithelialisation. The wound-healing phase of inflammation is thus curtailed (since re-epithelialisation stops further evaporative water loss from the wound surface, signalling that wound healing is complete) and the outcomes excellent, with expedited scar maturation leading to an almost invisible repair after a few months for the majority of patients. **Figure 2** is a photograph of a mixed depth arm burn.

However, in common with all wounds, the phenotype of individual patients can proffer a predilection for substandard scarring, despite appropriate initial burn management. Individuals with a history of hypertrophic or keloid scarring, autoimmune or immunocompromised disorders and collagen or healing impairments may progress to suboptimal scarring [16]. It is for this reason that burn services have

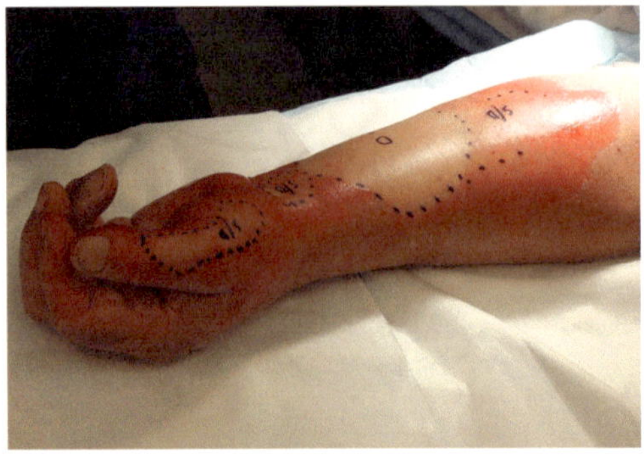

Figure 2.
Illustrating burn depth: D is deep dermal, S/D superficial/deep junction. The S/D areas have a variable healing time that is dependent on patient and operative factors.

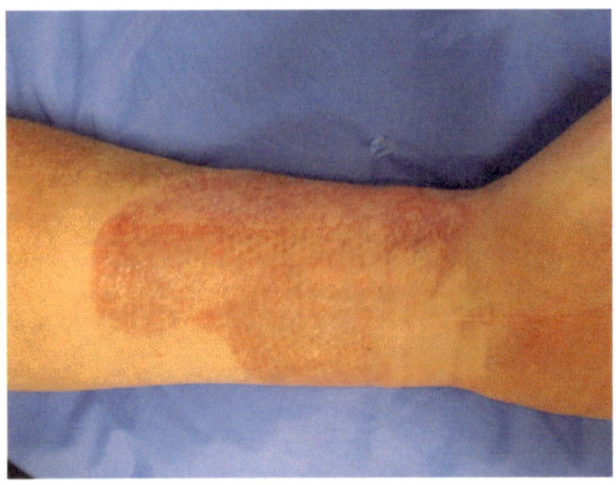

Figure 3.
Meshed split skin graft to forearm 6 weeks post-grafting and demonstrating good healing.

been an early adopter of the multidisciplinary approach, with an emphasis on scar management by occupational therapists and physiotherapists, once wound healing has been achieved [17]. Scar modulation techniques include pressure garments, topical silicone materials, massage, moisturising and steroid injection and will be further discussed in this chapter.

3.2 Deep dermal and full-thickness burns

A burn that is significantly deep enough to lack the capacity to heal quickly must undergo prolonged healing by secondary intention and result in pathological scarring [18], determined by a prolonged inflammatory phase and an abnormal proliferative phase. The resultant granulation of the wound bed followed by migration of myofibroblasts and contraction results in unstable scars. The epidermis will only bridge 5 mm across a wound; therefore contraction is inevitable. Unstable and contracted scars are particularly problematic. Contracture across joints will result in reduced movement and function. Contractures of the skin of the head and neck can risk vision (via ectropion and corneal exposure, desiccation and ulceration) and ability to feed (microstomia and lower lip contractures). The microtrauma that consistently causes fissures in the epidermis of the pathological scar can result in recurrent episodes of infection, further inflammation and thus further scarring.

Since the natural history of secondary intention healing of deep burns results in suboptimal scarring, the goal of burn surgery is to abort this process in favour of early physiological wound closure and healing, followed by scar management and rehabilitation, in order to achieve the best functional outcome [19]. The traditional mainstay of this process is the split skin graft, harvested from non-burned skin, which may be meshed to different ratios to enable wider wound coverage. **Figure 3** shows a meshed SSG on the forearm 6 weeks following excision and grafting.

If early physiological closure is our goal, the importance of early and accurate assessment of burn depth is vital. Identification of deeper burn and initiation of early surgical intervention significantly improve function, aesthetic appearance and return for the patient to normal daily activity.

4. Size of the burn

Information regarding burn depth is complimented by knowledge of the size (surface area) of the burn. This is estimated as a percentage of the total body surface area injured (%TBSA) and is an essential factor in determining scar outcome. A small area of full-thickness burn can be reliably treated with early excision and immediate skin grafting. The inflammatory reaction to the burn is localised to the affected area; donor site for the split skin graft can be reliably taken from a non-cosmetic area. Large donor site availability even gives us options for better 'colour-matching' our skin graft! Early scar therapy can begin once the graft has taken and is robust.

However, as burn size increases, the challenges of treatment increase accordingly. Three burn-area percentages are considered important for burn surgeons: 20, 50 and 80% TBSA. At 20% TBSA, intravenous fluid resuscitation is routinely initiated, and the effect of the burn inflammatory response ceases to be localised to the burn area and has systemic consequences. The resultant fluid shifts and loss from the circulation are thus markedly more significant and, if untreated, result in burn shock with cardiac and renal consequences [20, 21]. At 50% TBSA, the burn area usually exceeds the available donor site area (since we do not harvest grafts from the unburned face, neck, palms of hands or soles of feet). Strategies for wound closure become important. At burn sizes just in excess of 50% TBSA, this might merely involve skin graft meshing at a higher ratio (say 1:3, rather than 1:1.5). At greater burn sizes, serial grafting may be necessary and should be planned to heal pivotal areas first (hands, face, neck, major joints, etc.). Additionally, dermal temporising materials are purchased (at great financial cost), and cultured skin equivalents (usually simply epidermal cells, keratinocytes; but occasionally composite cultured tissues) are prepared by those services capable of such technology. Basically, to facilitate skin closure for burns above 50% TBSA, almost all of the unburned skin must be harvested, often repeatedly. Since the dermal component of the skin graft donor site cannot undergo regeneration (and donor sites therefore being progressively 'thinner' after each graft), we tend to take thinner split skin grafts (i.e. with less dermal component) to allow a greater number of graft harvests. The combination of being thinner and more widely meshed reduces functional and aesthetic outcome because such grafts contract more, and more rapidly, than thicker, less/unmeshed graft. Thus, the techniques involved guarantee that the patient with the biggest burn who really needs the best possible outcome to regain important components of their pre-injury existence survives with the poorest functional, aesthetic and symptomatic outcome possible and illustrates why skin burns of the same depth demonstrate poorer scarring outcomes as burn surface area increases. This is further complicated by the fact that these patients are at higher risk of multi-organ dysfunction [21].

Finally, full-thickness burns ≥80% TBSA in adults often prove fatal. These overwhelming skin injuries leave very little or no unburned areas to allow even serial wound repair and are frequently accompanied by smoke inhalation and other co-injuries. Such injuries are classified as unsurvivable in the majority of burn units [22–24], receiving palliative, comfort care only prior to death. For patients who do survive these devastating injuries, long-term scarring issues are daunting, and return to useful function is extremely challenging.

5. Special anatomical areas of consideration

In addition to burn depth and size, burns (and subsequently scarring) to certain 'special' areas of the body have the potential to be not only functionally disabling but also psychosocially disastrous, requiring immediate or early reconstruction.

5.1 Face, neck and hands

The face, neck and hands are areas of extreme functional and aesthetic importance. If reconstruction requires grafting, the best functional and cosmetic outcomes are generated by thicker, unmeshed (sheet) split skin grafts. In the patient with significant burns, this requires a large proportion of the available donor sites to cover relatively small surface area defects, whilst bigger areas are left un-grafted. Protecting the ocular globes and ensuring oral competence are important, but reconstruction of the eyelids and lips is challenging. In the non-burn, or small isolated burn situation, small full-thickness grafts or flaps are often used for such reconstructions, resources sadly lacking in the major burn patient. It is thus crucial during the management of facial burns to identify those areas capable of healing spontaneously, bearing in mind that the deeper adnexal structures in facial skin often allow even burns which appear deep to heal without intervention. The best course of action is often to allow the face to heal spontaneously as much as possible and then plan appropriate reconstruction for scarred areas [25, 26]. The neck is prioritised for early grafting not only for function but also to allow for tracheostomy placement as severely burned patients may require prolonged ICU stay and ventilation. Full-thickness burns on the dorsal aspect of the hands are grafted to allow early mobilisation and return to function, and early intervention by occupational and physiotherapists will improve outcome [27]. A good result for the hand dorsum is important since these scars are constantly in the field of vision and poor results are associated with post-injury depression. The glabrous skin on the palm and areas of partial thickness burn are routinely allowed a 'trial of life' to allow preservation of this highly specialised skin [28].

5.2 Joints

Split thickness skin graft heal with a variable degree of secondary contraction dependant on their thickness. When a graft is placed over a joint, in particular the elbow and knee, the effect of contracture is reduced range of movement and scar instability. This contracture is much less significant than if the burn had been left to heal by secondary intention, but subsequent scar management requires intensive occupational therapy and physiotherapy to regain and maintain range of motion. Contractures are more likely to occur in the more severe burns, those caused by flame and those in children and females, and burns affecting the neck skin (due to the presence of the platysma) and the upper limb. The prevalence at discharge has been reported as 38–54% [18].

6. Scarring issues peculiar to burns

Burn healing can result in hypertrophic scarring, with functional disability and debilitating symptoms including dysaethesia, pain and itch. It is estimated that up to 70% of burn patients will have some evidence of scar hypertrophy [29].

In addition to optimal surgical management, scar modulation measures include reducing tension across the scar, the provision of taping, hydration and ultraviolet (UV) protection of early scar tissue. Silicone sheeting, or gel, is universally considered as the first-line prophylactic and treatment option for hypertrophic or keloid scars. The efficacy and safety of this gold-standard, non-invasive therapy have been demonstrated in many clinical studies [30]. Hypertrophy is managed by aggressive scar modulation including pressure garments, silicone therapy and moisturising and massage. These interventions are all proven to be beneficial although the exact mechanisms remain to be elucidated [31]. Pressure garments may be indicated for more widespread scarring associated with burn. Both pressure garments and silicone therapy can be referred to as scar modulation. Massage and moisturising are often described as 'softening' scars, most likely due to the reorientation of collagen fibres. An ideal moisturiser should be one that is conducive to scar maturation, is non- or minimally irritant, prevents skin drying, minimises trans-epidermal water loss and has no negative effect on barrier function [32].

The symptomatic manifestations of suboptimal scarring are particularly difficult to manage, particularly pain and itch, which are often interlinked and not uncommon [33]. Intractable itch is challenging as the symptoms are subjective and the treatment is multimodal with no 'magic bullet' to prevent or ameliorate it.

Pain control and analgesia is vitally important, particularly during dressing changes, and pharmacological management facilitated by experts in pain medicine is essential. Pain control is also essential in order to deliver effective rehabilitation.

Newer therapies, such as music therapy and virtual reality distraction, are useful adjuncts to clinical psychology input which provides insight into a patient's reaction to and ability to cope with pain [34, 35].

7. Shifting the paradigm

The case for early total excision has been demonstrated in the literature [36, 37], and temporary wound closure is necessary due to lack of donor sites; it is in this area that skin substitutes have been developed to facilitate wound coverage. Cadaver allograft skin has been used extensively as a 'passive' temporiser (holding the wound bed without improving its quality), but access to, and availability of, this resource are highly variable [38].

The dermal matrix strategy sought to redress some of these issues [39]. Scaffolds of varying composition have been employed as 'active' temporisers, allowing autologous tissue ingrowth to form a 'neo-dermis' which improves the wound bed for subsequent definitive closure. Such dermal matrices have historically been a combination of synthetic and biological materials (e.g. Integra® Dermal Regeneration Template consists of a network of cross-linked, bovine Type I collagen supported by shark fin-derived chondroitin-6-sulphate glycosaminoglycan (GAG), physiologically closed with a bonded silicone pseudo-epidermis) [40]. The biological aspect can cause issues as burn patients are frequently immunocompromised and rapidly become bacterially colonised, and these biological components have neither intrinsic antimicrobial properties nor are sufficiently rapidly neovascularised to be afforded the innate immune protection provided by a blood supply. As a result, they may be susceptible to infection [41]. The production of these materials is also complex and time-consuming, making such materials costly. However, the use of Integra® and similar materials has been pivotal in saving life and improving outcome over several decades [40].

Since the scaffold supports ingrowth into the spaces within it, it can be argued that it can be composed of any biodegradable material as long as it is biocompatible, bio-tolerated and safe (not cytotoxic, carcinogenic or teratogenic). The development of a completely synthetic biodegradable temporising matrix (BTM) developed from a biodegradable polyurethane is proof in point. BTM is implanted into the wound created after burn excision and integrates by facilitating fibroblast invasion, collagen deposition and neovascular ingrowth to also form a neo-dermal analogue [42–45]. This takes between 3 and 9 weeks, dependant on the quality of the wound bed. The bonded, non-biodegradable polyurethane outer 'seal' (or pseudo-epidermis, since it prevents evaporative water loss) ensures the wound is physiologically 'closed'.

The integration period allows for initial stabilisation and improvement in physiological status prior to administering insults such as skin graft harvesting. In all cases, the patient is off the ICU before skin grafting commences. The improved neo-dermal wound bed receives graft more readily, with negligible graft loss, and with a significantly reduced mesh pattern where meshed graft has been employed [46–48]. This phenomenon has also been observed with collagen-based matrices [40].

The aim of burn reconstruction, in common with all aspects of plastic surgery, is to replace 'like with like', and, as such, the standard treatment of excised burns has been the split skin graft (despite the fact that the autograft is a long way from replacing what has been lost!). The major hindrance to this approach is the lack of donor site, the necessity to serially re-harvest donor sites and the resultant suboptimal scarring from using thin, widely meshed autograft. The future of burn surgery lies in creating composite tissue from the patients' own skin cells, or stem cell progenitors, as a means to abolish the need for extensive donor sites [49]. The preparation of composite tissues takes several weeks, and thus the use of 'active' temporising skin substitutes is a fundamental first step.

Cultured skin, like autograft, has the advantage of being 'self' and thus accepted immunologically by the patient, as long as the carrier for the cell culture is immunologically inert [50].

8. Late scar management

Scars can take up to 24 months to mature fully. This is a window during which scar modulation can be effective and should persist in some form throughout this period. However, if a scar is significantly problematic (in terms of function, aesthetics or intolerable symptoms), early surgical scar revision may be necessary.

Scar revision can be broadly divided into three groups: scar resurfacing, scar excision or scar lengthening/reorientation. Scar resurfacing modalities include dermabrasion, microneedling and laser therapy. Depending on scar size, its excision can be followed by direct closure, split or full-thickness skin grafting, local flaps, free tissue transfer or a combination of dermal matrix and graft. Scar lengthening often involves incising the scar and reorientating the scar banding, usually by geometrically designed local flaps. The main reasons for performing scar revision are to resurface unstable scarring, improve movement at joints or to improve cosmesis [51].

However, it is the senior author's opinion that the requirement for secondary scar revision is lessened if the appropriate primary reconstruction is performed in a timely manner combined with early adjunctive scar management therapy.

9. Conclusion

In summary, the important tenets for the optimal management of burn scarring include:

- Accurate burn depth and burn size assessment
- Immediate/early burn eschar excision and rapid wound closure with either immediate skin grafting or staged with temporising skin substitutes plus skin grafting and/or cultured skin
- Peculiar consideration for burns affecting the special areas: face and neck, hands and joints
- Immediate scar management and mobilisation utilising therapists
- Later scar management including resurfacing and excision.

Conflict of interest

Professor John Greenwood would like to disclose that he holds shares in PolyNovo Biomaterials Pty Ltd. (the manufacturer of the NovoSorb™ foam and BTM™ device).

Dr. Lindsay Damkat-Thomas has no conflict of interest to declare.

Author details

Lindsay Damkat-Thomas* and John Edward Greenwood
Adult Burn Centre, Royal Adelaide Hospital, Adelaide, Australia

*Address all correspondence to: ldamkat@gmail.com

References

[1] The experience of life after burn injury: A new bodily awareness. Journal of Advanced Nursing. 2008;**64**(3):278-286

[2] Gille J, Schmidt T, Dragu A, Emich D, Hilbert-Carius P, Kremer T, et al. Electrical injury—A dual center analysis of patient characteristics, therapeutic specifics and outcome predictors. Scandinavian Journal of Trauma, Resuscitation and Emergency Medicine. 2018;**26**(1):43

[3] Shih JG, Shahrokhi S, Jeschke MG. Review of adult electrical burn injury outcomes worldwide: An analysis of low-voltage vs high-voltage electrical injury. Journal of Burn Care & Research. 2017;**38**(1):e293-e298

[4] Toon MH, Maybauer MO, Greenwood JE, Maybauer DM, Fraser JF. Management of acute smoke inhalation injury. Critical Care and Resuscitation. 2010;**12**(1):53-61

[5] Tan Chor Lip H, Tan JH, Thomas M, Imran FH, Azmah Tuan Mat TN. Survival analysis and mortality predictors of hospitalized severe burn victims in a Malaysian burns intensive care unit. Burns Trauma. 2019;7:3

[6] Friedstat JS, Ryan CM, Gibran N. Outcome metrics after burn injury: From patient-reported outcome measures to value-based health care. Clinics in Plastic Surgery. 2017;**44**(4):911-915. DOI: 10.1016/j.cps.2017.05.023

[7] Hawkins HK, Pereira CT. Pathophysiology of the burn scar. In: Total Burn Care. 3rd ed. Philadelphia, Pennsylvania, USA: Elsevier; 2007. pp. 608-617. ISBN: 978-1-4160-3274-8

[8] Clark RA. Basics of cutaneous wound repair. The Journal of Dermatologic Surgery and Oncology. 1993;**19**:693-706

[9] Ross R, Odland G. Human wound repair. II Inflammatory cells, epithelial-mesenchymal interrelations, and fibrogenesis. The Journal of Cell Biology. 1968;**39**:152-168

[10] Clark RA. Biology of dermal wound repair. Dermatologic Clinics. 1993;**11**:647-666

[11] Gabbiani D, Ryan GD, Majino G. Presence of modified fibroblasts in granulation tissue and their possible role in wound contraction. Experientia. 1971;**27**:549-550

[12] Greenwood JE, Kavanagh S, Mackie P. Revisiting protocols for burn injury management. International Journal of Care Pathways. 2010;**14**:88-95

[13] Greenwood JE, Clausen J, Kavanagh S. Experience with biobrane: Uses and caveats for success. Eplasty. 2009;**9**:243-255

[14] Stenn KS, Depalma L. In: RAF C, editor. Re-epithelialization, The Molecular and Cellular Biology of Wound Repair. New York: Plenum; 1996. pp. 321-335

[15] Daly TJ. The repair phase of wound healing—Re-epithelialization and contraction. In: Kloth LC, McCullough J, Feedar JS, EDS Wound Healing. Philadelphia: FA Davies; 1990. pp. 14-30

[16] Burd A, Huang L. Hypertrophic response and keloid diathesis: Two very different forms of scar. Plastic and Reconstructive Surgery. 2005;**116**:150e-157e

[17] Herndon DN, Bleakley PE. Team work for total burn care. In: Total Burn Care. 3rd ed. Philadelphia, Pennsylvania, USA: Elsevier; 2007. pp. 9-13. ISBN: 978-1-4160-3274-8

[18] Oosterwijk AM, Mouton LJ, Schouten H, Disseldorp LM, van der Schans CP, Nieuwenhuis MK. Prevalence of scar contractures after burn: A systematic review. Burns. 2017;**43**(1):41-49

[19] Richard R, Santos-Lozada AR, Dewey WS, Chung KK. Profile of patients without burn scar contracture development. Journal of Burn Care & Research. 2017;**38**(1):e62-e69

[20] Serio-Melvin ML, Salinas J, Chung KK, Collins C, Graybill JC, Harrington DT, et al. Burn shock and resuscitation: Proceedings of a symposium conducted at the meeting of the American Burn Association, Chicago, IL, 21 April 2015. Journal of Burn Care & Research. 2017;**38**(1):e423-e431

[21] Rae L, Fidler P, Gibran N. The physiologic basis of burn shock and the need for aggressive fluid resuscitation. Critical Care Clinics. 2016;**32**(4):491-505

[22] J Partain NS, Subramanian M, Hodgman EI, Isbell CL, Wolf SE, Arnoldo BD, et al. End-of-life care after geriatric burns at a verified level I burn center. Palliative Medicine. 2016;**19**(12):1275-1280

[23] Mahar PD, Wasiak J, Cleland H, Paul E, Loke SY, Fong HC, et al. Clinical differences between major burns patients deemed survivable and non-survivable on admission. Injury. 2015;**46**(5):870-873

[24] Greenwood JE. Development of patient pathways for the surgical management of burn injury. ANZ Journal of Surgery. 2006;**76**:805-811

[25] Friedstat JS, Klein MB. Acute management of facial burns. Clinics in Plastic Surgery. 2009;**36**(4):653-660

[26] Clayton NA, Ward EC, Maitz PK. Orofacial contracture management outcomes following partial thickness facial burns. Burns. 2015;**41**(6):1291-1297

[27] Sorkin M, Cholok D, Levi B. Scar management of the burned hand. Hand Clinics. 2017;**33**(2):305-315

[28] van Zuijlen PP, Kreis RW, Vloemans AF, Groenevelt F, Mackie DP. The prognostic factors regarding long-term functional outcome of full-thickness hand burns. Burns. 1999;**25**(8):709-714

[29] Bombaro KM, Engrav LH, Carrougher GJ, et al. What is the prevalence of hypertrophic scarring following burns? Burns. 2003;**29**:299-302

[30] Monstrey S, Middelkoop E, Vranckx JJ, Bassetto F, Ziegler UE, Meaume S, et al. Updated scar management practical guidelines: Non-invasive and invasive measures. Journal of Plastic Reconstructive & Aesthetic Surgery. 2014;**67**(8):1017-1025

[31] Tredget EE, Shupp JW, Schneider JC. Scar management following burn injury. Journal of Burn Care & Research. 2017;**38**(3):146-147. DOI: 10.1097/BCR.0000000000000548

[32] Klotz T, Kurmis R, Munn Z, Heath K, Greenwood J. Moisturisers in scar management following burn: A survey report. Burns. 2017;**43**(5):965-972

[33] Mauck MC, Smith J, Liu AY, Jones SW, Shupp JW, Villard MA, et al. Chronic pain and itch are common, morbid sequelae among individuals who receive tissue autograft after major thermal burn injury. The Clinical Journal of Pain. 2017;**33**(7):627-634

[34] Hoffman HG, Chambers GT, Meyer WJ 3rd, Arceneaux LL, Russell WJ, Seibel EJ, et al. Virtual reality as an adjunctive non-pharmacologic analgesic for acute burn pain during medical

procedures. Annals of Behavioral Medicine. 2011;**41**(2):183-191

[35] Najafi Ghezeljeh T, Mohades Ardebili F, Rafii F. The effects of massage and music on pain, anxiety and relaxation in burn patients: Randomized controlled clinical trial. Burns. 2017;**43**(5):1034-1104

[36] Herndon DN, Barrow RE, Rutan RL, Rutan TC, Desai MH, Abston S. A comparison of conservative versus early excision. Therapies in severely burned patients. Annals of Surgery. 1989;**209**(5):547-552

[37] Janzekovic Z. A new concept in the early excision and immediate grafting of burns. The Journal of Trauma. 1970;**10**(12):1103-1108

[38] Cleland H, Wasiak J, Dobson H, Paul M, Pratt G, Paul E, et al. Clinical application and viability of cryopreserved cadaveric skin allografts in severe burn: A retrospective analysis. Burns. 2014;**40**(1):61-66

[39] Branski LK, Herndon DN, Pereira C, Mlcak RP, Celis MM, Lee JO, et al. Longitudinal assessment of Integra in primary burn management: A randomized pediatric clinical trial. Critical Care Medicine. 2007;**35**(11):2615-2623

[40] Heimbach DM, Warden GD, Luterman A, Jordan MH, Ozobia N, Ryan CM, et al. Multicenter postapproval clinical trial of Integra dermal regeneration template for burn treatment. Journal of Burn Care & Rehabilitation. 2003;**24**(1):42-48

[41] Bargues L, Boyer S, Leclerc T, Duhamel P, Bey E. Incidence and microbiology of infectious complications with the use of artificial skin Integra in burns. Annales de Chirurgie Plastique et Esthétique. 2009;**54**(6):533-539

[42] Li A, Dearman BL, Crompton KE, Moore TG, Greenwood JE. Evaluation of a novel biodegradable polymer for the generation of a dermal matrix. Journal of Burn Care & Research. 2009;**30**(4):717-728

[43] Greenwood JE, Li A, Dearman B, Moore TG. Evaluation of NovoSorb™ novel biodegradable polymer for the generation of a dermal matrix. Part 1: In-vitro studies. Wound Practice & Research. 2010;**18**(1):14-22

[44] Greenwood JE, Li A, Dearman B, Moore TG. Evaluation of NovoSorb™ novel biodegradable polymer for the generation of a dermal matrix. Part 2: In-vivo studies. Wound Practice & Research. 2010;**18**(1):24-34

[45] Greenwood JE, Dearman BL. Split-skin graft application over an integrating, biodegradable temporising polymer matrix: Immediate and delayed. Journal of Burn Care & Research. 2012;**33**(1):7-19

[46] Greenwood JE, Schmitt BJ, Wagstaff MJD. Experience with a synthetic bilayer biodegradable temporising matrix in significant burn injury. Burns Open. 2018;**2**:17-34

[47] Greenwood JE, Wagstaff MJD, Rooke M, Caplash Y. Reconstruction of extensive calvarial exposure after major burn injury in two stages using a biodegradable polyurethane matrix. Eplasty. 2016;**16**:151-160

[48] Greenwood JE, Wagstaff MJD. The use of biodegradable polyurethane in the development of dermal scaffolds. Chapter 22. In: Cooper SL, Guan J, editors. Advances in Polyurethane Biomaterials. Duxford, UK: Woodhead Publishing Series in Biomaterials, (Elsevier Inc.); 2016. ISBN: 978-0-08-100614-6

[49] Greenwood JE. The evolution of acute burn care—Retiring the

split skin graft. Annals of the Royal College of Surgeons of England. 2017;**99**(6):432-438

[50] Dearman BL, Stefani K, Li A, Greenwood JE. "Take" of a polymer-based autologous cultured composite "skin" on an integrated temporizing dermal matrix: Proof of concept. Journal of Burn Care & Research. 2013;**34**(11):151-160

[51] Finnerty CC, Jeschke MG, Branski LK, Barret JP, Dziewulski P, Herndon DN. Hypertrophic scarring: The greatest unmet challenge after burn injury. Lancet. 2016;**388**(10052):1427-1436

Section 3

Electrical Burns

Chapter 3

The Specificities of Electrical Burn Healing

Iyadh Ghorbel, Slim Moalla, Amal Abid, Amir Karra and Khalil Ennouri

Abstract

Electrical burns are a major cause of bodily harm due to the mechanism and effect of the lesions. This prompts us to study these lesions and their management in order to reduce the morbidity caused by this type of accident. In the event of an electric chock accident, the treatment is medico-surgical and is composed of two main phases: acute phase when general treatment is essential and subacute phase when local treatment is implemented. The study shows that conventional emergency decompression does not appear to reduce the amputation rate, the use of local and locoregional flaps in the initial phase (<21 days) carries a significant risk of suffering and necrosis, and also antithrombotic prevention or the use of flaps does not seem to have an impact on healing delays.

Keywords: burns, electrical, fasciotomy, antithrombotic, flap, healing time

1. Introduction

Electric burns are known for its devastating effects, leading to significant morbidity and mortality, especially as it often affects young adults of working age [1–7]. The lesions are often due to direct contact with the current, which during its passage through the body will cause tissue damage of varying severity depending on the voltage, the exposure time, and the tissue resistance [3, 8]. Low voltage burns (<1000 V) often cause local lesions, whereas high voltage burns (>1000 V) lead to extensive destruction of deep structures and systemic effects [9]. Advances in medical resuscitation have made it possible to increase the survival rate of electrified patients. However, the surgical management of electrical burns is controversial. Opinions are still discussed between early and wide excision with immediate reconstruction and late iterative excision and subsequent reconstruction based on several plastic surgery procedures [10].

2. Injury mechanism

2.1 The characteristics of electricity

The electric current is defined by:

1. Its intensity that corresponds to the electric charge carried by the electrons crossing a section of circuit during a second. It is measured in amperes denoted as A

2. Its voltage that corresponds to the circulation of the electric field along an electrical circuit measured in volts and denoted as V.

The injuries induced by the electric current thus depend on the voltage, the intensity, the contact time (T), and the resistance encountered expressed in R.

Four main mechanisms are evoked before any electric shock accident:

1. Depolarization lesions: they are due to the direct action of the current on the human cell whatever its type. It can induce a direct lesion of the nervous, cardiac, or muscular cells, which can cause cardio-respiratory arrest. In this case, we speak of an electrocution accident. The depolarization effect is a function of the current intensity.

2. Heat-induced lesions: produced by the passage of the current according to the resistance of the tissues governed by the Joule law: J = I2.R.t or U.I.R.t.

   Thus, the higher the tissue resistance is, the more heat will be emitted and the more serious the lesions will be. Note that fluid environments, nerves, blood, and vessels are low resistance tissues that emit little heat during the passage of electric current and lesions will be minimal. However, the skin (mainly the stratum corneum) and the bone tissues are of high resistance and emit a lot of heat, which will cause lesions in the tissue cells in addition to a devastating action on the surrounding tissues like the muscles [11].

   On the other hand, depending on the voltage, we can distinguish two types of lesions:

   Low voltage burns, when the voltage is less than 1000 V. In this case, the lesions are often less serious but where the intensity can sometimes cause significant lesions.

   - High voltage burns, when the voltage is over 1000 V. In this case, the lesions are most often serious.

   - Finally, the contact time contributes to the severity of the lesions: the longer it is prolonged, the more serious the lesions will be.

3. Electric flash: these are thermal burns that can be observed during an electric shock accident and are secondary to the spark that can occur during contact with the electricity [11, 12]

4. Electric arc: it is a rare phenomenon but which must not be neglected. Thus in some cases when the voltage is very high, there can be an attack without direct contact with the current. The electric jump distance is 2–3 m per 10,000 V [11]. This high voltage generated remotely can cause real skin and muscle damage. It has been calculated that the heat produced can vary from 2000 to 20,000°C [11].

2.2 Anatomopathology

In front of an electric burn, practitioner has always to look for the entry point and the exit point, which will make it possible to imagine the path of the current and thus evaluate the severity of the damage and lesions.

The skin is the first organ affected, and then the current follows through variable and unpredictable paths depending on the degree of resistance encountered.

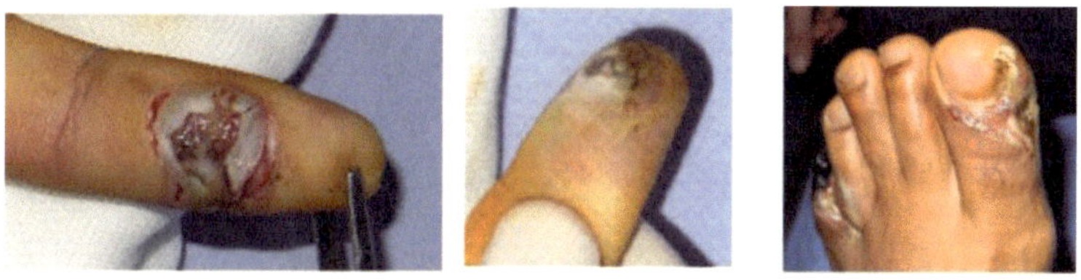

Figure 1.
Entry point in fingers. Exit point in toes.

Finally, it will go out of the body through the skin at a zone in contact with the ground or another external element.

At the entry point is a marble colored or whitish area, charred, insensitive and does not bleed when scarification is done (**Figure 1**). Its size is very small in area ranging from a few millimeters to centimeters. The most serious damage is deep. In fact under a dry skin, a high voltage current can generate a heat of more than 1000°C [11]. At the exit point, there is a small area of white and gray necrosis.

The hands and the feet constitute, respectively, the sites of predilections of entry and the exit of the electricity. The dominant side is most often reached during electrical burns [13–15]. Moreover, in the electric burn, the cutaneous lesion is not the accurate reflection of the extent of the underlying lesions related to the passage of the current. Burnt body surface is often small with percentages not exceeding 20% [16, 17].

The different tissues and organs can undergo lesions of variable severity that may be due to the direct action of electricity on the human cell or indirect by the effect of heat released depending on the tissue resistance.

On the other hand, the lesions can be giving extensive necrosis of the tissues, immediately or in the upcoming days as a result of the complications caused by the passage of the current such that:

1. The progressive devascularization of muscles and skin by thrombosis due to the direct action of the current on the vascular wall [18, 19] more or less associated with hypercoagulability.

2. Compartment syndrome: increase of the intra compartmental pressure > 28 mmHg.

3. Multi-resistant bacterial infections aggravating the lesions.

3. Epidemiological profile

Most series have reported an average age of 30.2 years [3, 12, 20, 21]. The prevalence of injury in the third decade may be due to occupation [12, 22, 23]. Mashreky et al. [21] have shown that the relative risk of having an electric burn is higher in men than in women. According to Dega et al. [24], 91% of electric burn victims are manual workers. In addition, the lesion most often affects the upper part of the trunk and the upper limb.

Most frequently, it is a domestic accident [21, 22, 25]. This is often due to inexcusable negligence of security measures [21]. Many authors [2, 10, 21] reported the association of household accidents with low-voltage burns, while work and public road accidents are linked with high-voltage burns.

4. Patient management

In the event of an electric chock accident, the treatment is medico-surgical and is composed of two main phases.

4.1 Acute phase

4.1.1 General treatment

The patient must be conditioned and a solute infusion must be started. It is necessary first of all to eliminate a lesion which can be lethal: essentially cardiac depolarization disorders as it can lead to cardiac arrest (electrocution) and/or head trauma by falling from height or projection during electrification accident. In the case of polytrauma, a body scan must be performed urgently.

About 10–20% of patients arriving at hospital show electrocardiographic disturbances such as supraventricular tachycardia (SVT), right bundle-branch block, arrhythmia, and nonspecific ST segment disturbances at the ECG [11]. On the other hand, the electrified patient is vulnerable to having a myocardial infarction given the lesions created by the current at the level of the vessel wall and the formation of thrombosis. The dosage of cardiac enzymes (troponin) must be systematic and recontrolled. Thus, most authors agree on the need to introduce initial heparin therapy, in order to minimize these thromboembolic risks [26].

An evaluation of renal function by serum creatinine determination and hourly diuresis monitoring as well as the determination of muscle enzymes (CPK and LDH) can detect possible acute functional or organic renal failure by tubular necrosis [7].

4.1.2 Local treatment

In electric shock accidents, depending on the series, 9.2–54% of the victims may require the urgent realization of a fasciotomy and/or escharotomy [10, 16, 27]. This could be explained by the localization of the entry wound as well as the aggressiveness of the electric passage.

The realization of a fasciotomy in emergency is guided by the presence or not of a compartment syndrome and the monitoring of the intra-compartmental pressure which must not exceed 28 mmHg. Fasciotomy timing (immediate or secondary) and technique (total or selective) are subject to controversy. Previously, it was recommended to perform systematically a total fasciotomy in front of any electrical burn of the limbs. Recent studies, however, advocate selective and nonimmediate decompression to preserve the tissues and reduce the rate of amputations [10].

Moreover, during electrical burns, 20–30% of patients undergo amputation [16, 20, 24] with a statistically significant relationship between "the type of voltage and amputation" and "the high voltage and the comorbidity" [16, 28, 29]. It is often an amputation of a limb or limb segment [29]. It is necessary to respect the rules of amputation (suitable level, burial of the nerves) and a stump of good quality guaranteeing an adequate prosthesis without complications (**Figure 2**). Amputation is rarely done urgently, except in case of irreversible distal ischemia or massive necrosis by direct attack with hemodynamic repercussions that can be life threatening.

4.2 Subacute phase

Once the hemodynamic state is stabilized and the critical course is surpassed, the management is focused on the prevention of any complications and their

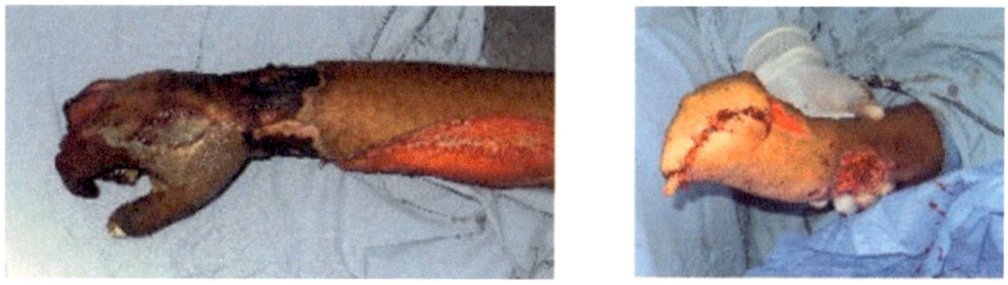

Figure 2.
Hand necrosis. Amputation.

treatment, and on the healing of various lesions, modality and deadlines remain controversial.

Some authors believe that tissue damage is fully established immediately and that there is no change in necrosis and thus advocates early and wide excision with immediate free flap reconstruction [10, 13, 25]. This attitude reduces the rate of infectious complications, the time to heal, and the length of hospital stay [30].

Other authors believe that the damage is done in two stages in which the initial trauma is followed by progressive tissue necrosis essentially at the level of the deep muscular compartments [3, 10, 14], and thus that the evolutionary nature of these lesions requires iterative debridement with secondary reconstruction [31, 32].

In our practice, the first excision is performed on an average of 8 days after burns. Reconstruction will be immediate by autoplasty if there is exposure of bone, joint, nerve, or vascular element [7].

4.2.1 Healing modalities

Healing by secondary intention is the method of choice for many authors [11, 16]. The use of flaps, especially free flaps, is frequent compared to other etiologies of burns [20] and this which aims reducing morbidity. However, their vitality can be disrupted which questions the optimal moment of the reconstruction.

During the primary phase, the risk of necrosis is amplified and can reach up to 24% according to Sauerbier et al. [10, 33]. This phase has been described as a phase of vulnerability that lasts about 21 days and during which there is vascular instability that can compromise the vitality of the flap [10, 34]. Therefore, it is recommended to use the flap as far as possible from the electrified area [18] such as the groin flap and the latissimus dorsi flap [10].

Regional and local flaps are often used as an excellent means of coverage with lower morbidity and a similar success rate to free flaps [7, 24]. Moreover, the free flaps are used secondarily in case of necrosis or immediately in case of a large skin defect. We recommend using autoplasty during the secondary phase after delimitation of necrosis and stability of vascular lesions (**Figure 3**).

Perforator pedicled flaps are an important tool for reconstruction especially in small and average size skin defects. This kind of flaps permits “like by like” reconstruction using microsurgical nonmicrovascular flaps [35]. The main advantages of these flaps could be summarized as: no microsurgical sutures, no main vascular pedicles sacrifice, same surgical field, and shorter hospitalization time (**Figure 4**).

In deep burns with complete destruction of the dermis, the use of definitive skin substitutes (artificial dermis) aims at reconstructing a neodermis, in particular at the level of the functional zones, but it can also be used at limited tendon or osteoarticular exposures, subject to a well vascularized environment [31]. However, given their considerable cost, their use remains limited to burn centers that have such means.

The use of the vacuum-assisted closure (VAC) therapy after debridement has been described by some authors [36–38] who reported that this technique can

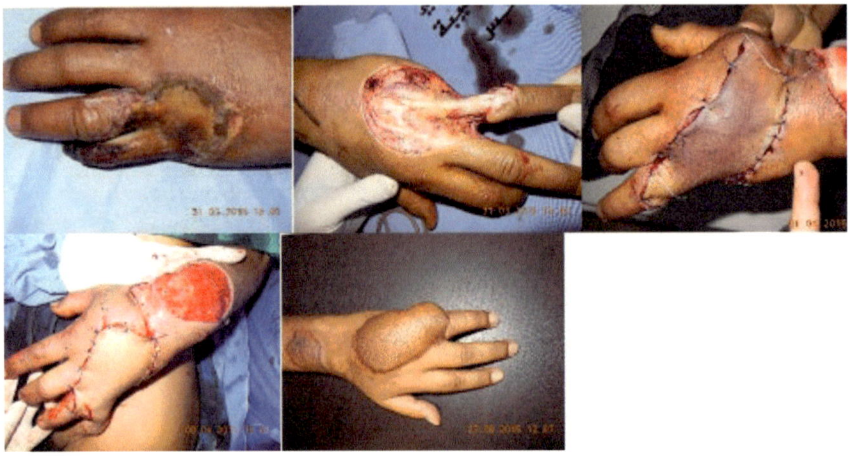

Figure 3.
Low voltage electric burn. Necrosis of the fifth finger. Excision 6 days after burn. Immediate coverage by local flap. Partial necrosis of the flap. Groin flap.

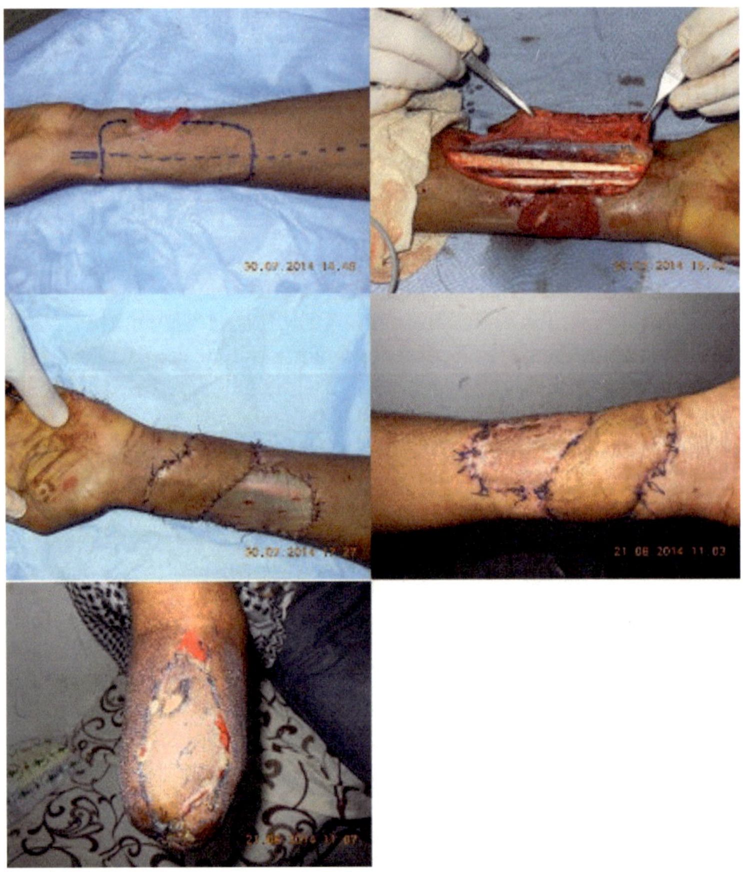

Figure 4.
High voltage electric burn. Radial artery perforator flap for the left upper limb. Right upper limb amputation.

reduce the frequency of dressing changes and the exposure time. The application of a VAC system requires that the debridement phase should be completed. It accelerates the granulation phase and shortens the duration of hospitalization. In addition, we preserve this technique with deep and small skin defects (**Figure 5**).

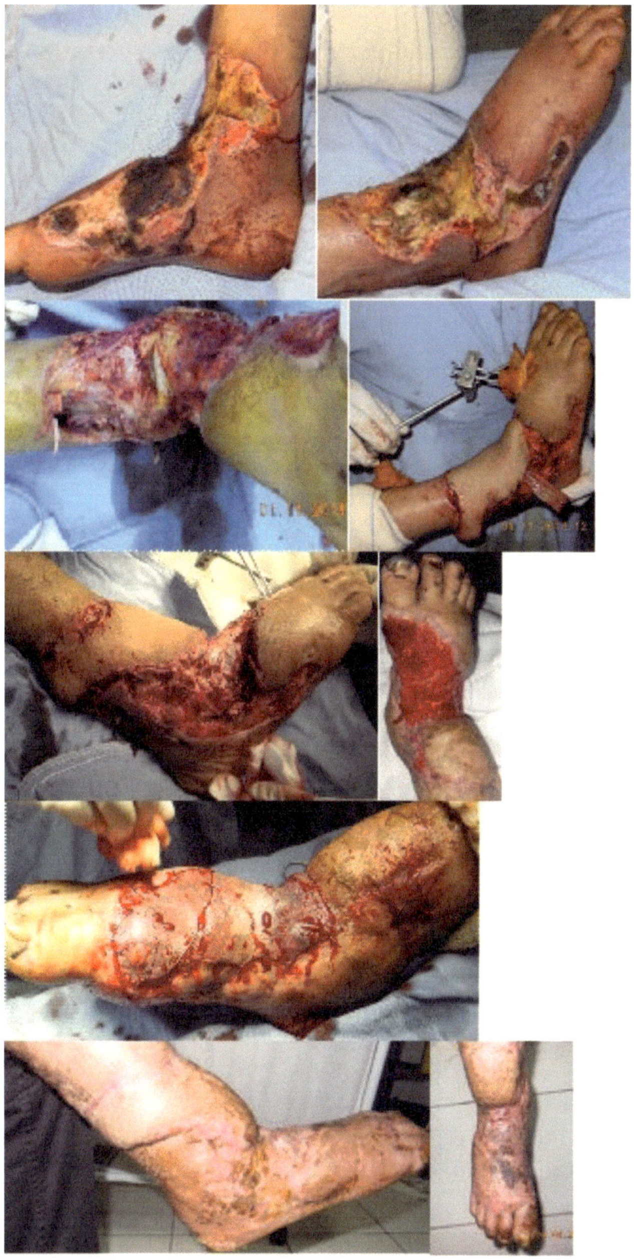

Figure 5.
High voltage electric burn. Excision 7 days after burn with osteoarticular exposition. Use of sural flap, vacuum-assisted closure therapy and skin grafting.

4.2.2 Healing time

The healing time does not depend on the total burn surface area (TBSA) or the healing modality (second intention or first intention). In our practice, it was found that, first, most patients who had flap cover healed beyond 1 month, and second, the flap cover in electrical burns, and despite its efficient functional and esthetic results, it prolongs the healing time. This is largely related to the severity of the initial lesions, lesions localization (joints and periorificial area), terrain, and infectious complications [7].

The mean healing time in our series was 48.91 ± 23.16 days with a median of 45 days [7]. However, most series reports the time of hospitalization during electric burns [2, 3, 39] which is 53.43 ± 31.73 days according to Lipovy et al. According to us, we think that the management of a burnt, electrical, or other, is not reduced to the period of hospitalization but extends to the healing of the various lesions. In most cases, this cannot be done entirely in hospital and, thus, many patients benefit from an external follow-up phase.

Most authors admit that high-voltage electrical burns heal late, compared with low-voltage burns, given the large amount of energy emitted by the tissue and the depth of the lesions [3].

However, there was no statistically significant relationship between the type of voltage and healing time or between the introduction of preventive, anti-thrombotic therapy, and the healing time. This can be explained by the small number of our patients' sample. In addition, as a specialized service, there has been a selection bias in our series since hospitalized patients are those with the most severe lesions even with low voltage current and require sophisticated healing processes [7].

4.3 Sequela

The majority of patients who have suffered an electric shock accident have more or less disabling sequela [20, 24, 40]. In fact, the voltage would predict neither the rate of the return to work nor the rate of neuropsychiatric sequela, and that the patients evolve in the same way in terms of sequela independently of the voltage of the causal current [41].

4.3.1 Cutaneous sequela

They are often described as keloid and hypertrophic scars, dyschromia, and skin retractions [7, 40]. In the initial phase, the treatment is medical (pressotherapy and silicone gel). Surgery will only be indicated after scar maturation except in cases of major functional repercussions.

4.3.2 Neurological sequela

Peripheral post-burn neurologic sequela are well documented nowadays and are both troublesome and disabling sequela for patients who have suffered from electrical burns [8, 24, 40, 42].

These sequela ranges from simple paresis with sensitivity disorder to total paralysis. They may appear early or late [43]. In all cases, it is necessary to wait for the delay of 1 year before drawing up the definitive state.

4.3.3 Osteoarticular sequela

The rate of osteoarticular sequela is around 30% according to most series [7, 24, 40]. In addition to the more or less extensive amputations, joint stiffness, dysplasia, and ankylosis can also be described.

4.4 Socio-economic impact

Electrical burns, whether high or low voltage, can have a significant socio-economic impact due to absenteeism and inability to work [41]. However, a comparative study showed that although electric burn patients remained more in hospital and had a higher rate of amputations, there was no difference in terms of return to work compared to thermal burns [44].

4.5 Psychological impact

Psychological impacts following an electrical burn are not as rare as one might think and add psychological morbidity associated with physical morbidity in these patients. Psychiatric morbidity is present in 28–78% of burns. However, the type of voltage and the initial pain do not appear to be related to psychological sequela [8, 43, 45].

5. Conclusion

Electrical burns are serious trauma that should be properly managed to avoid serious functional and life-threatening consequences. However, this management continues to be hampered by the lack of established guidelines unifying treatment and improving the prognosis.

Conflict of interest

The authors declare no "conflict of interest."

Author details

Iyadh Ghorbel*, Slim Moalla, Amal Abid, Amir Karra and Khalil Ennouri
Plastic, Aesthetic and Reconstructive Surgery Department, Habib Bourguiba Hospital, Sfax, Tunisia

*Address all correspondence to: iadh_ghorbel@medecinesfax.org

References

[1] Costagliola M. Principes généraux de la chirurgie reconstructrice des séquelles de brûlures. Annales de Chirurgie Plastique Esthétique. 2011;**56**(5):354-357

[2] Lipový B, Kaloudová Y, Ríhová H, Chaloupková Z, Kempný T, Suchanek I, et al. High voltage electrical injury: An 11-year single center epidemiological study. Annals of Burns and Fire Disasters. 2014;**27**(2):82-86

[3] Yagmur C. Electrical burns: Highlights from a 5-year retrospective analysis. Turkish Journal of Trauma and Emergency Surgery. 2015. Available from: http://www.tjtes.org/eng/jvi.aspx?pdir=travma&plng=eng&un=UTD-55491&look4=

[4] Haddad SY. Electrical burn–A four-year study. Annals of Burns and Fire Disasters. 2008;**21**(2):78-80

[5] Luz DP, Millan LS, Alessi MS, Uguetto WF, Paggiaro A, Gomez DS, et al. Electrical burns: A retrospective analysis across a 5-year period. Burns. 2009;**35**(7):1015-1019

[6] Vierhapper MF, Lumenta DB, Beck H, Keck M, Kamolz LP, Frey M. Electrical injury: A long-term analysis with review of regional differences. Annals of Plastic Surgery. 2011;**66**(1):43-46

[7] Ghorbel I, Abid A, Moalla S, Karra A, Nouri K. La particularité de cicatrisation des pertes de substance cutanées dans les brûlures électriques: Notre expérience. Annals of Burns and Fire Disasters. 2018;**31**(2):122-126

[8] Singerman J, Gomez M, Fish JS. Long-term sequelae of low-voltage electrical injury. Journal of Burn Care & Research. 2008;**29**(5):773-777

[9] Lee RC. Injury by electrical forces: Pathophysiology, manifestations, and therapy. Current Problems in Surgery. 1997;**34**(9):677-764

[10] Handschin AE, Vetter S, Jung FJ, Guggenheim M, Künzi W, Giovanoli P. A case-matched controlled study on high-voltage electrical injuries vs thermal burns. Journal of Burn Care & Research. 2009;**30**(3):400-407

[11] Échinard C, Latarjet J. Les brûlures. Issy-Les-Moulineaux: Masson; 2010

[12] El Bouyousfi J, Fejjal N, Belkacem R. Les brûlures électriques de la main chez l'enfant. Journal de Pédiatrie et de Puériculture. 2015;**28**(4):173-176

[13] Mazzetto-Betti KC, Amâncio ACG, Farina JA, Barros MEPM, Fonseca MCR. High-voltage electrical burn injuries: Functional upper extremity assessment. Burns. 2009;**35**(5):707-713

[14] Noble J, Gomez M, Fish JS. Quality of life and return to work following electrical burns. Burns. 2006;**32**(2):159-164

[15] Brych SB, Engrav LH, Rivara FP, Ptacek JT, Lezotte DC, Esselman PC, et al. Time off work and return to work rates after burns: Systematic review of the literature and a large two-center series. The Journal of Burn Care & Rehabilitation. 2001;**22**(6):401-405

[16] Salehi SH, Fatemi MJ, Aśadi K, Shoar S, Ghazarian AD, Samimi R. Electrical injury in construction workers: A special focus on injury with electrical power. Burns. 2014;**40**(2):300-304

[17] Kym D, Seo DK, Hur GY, Lee JW. Epidemiology of electrical injury: Differences between low- and high-voltage electrical injuries during a 7-year study period in South Korea. Scandinavian Journal of Surgery. 2015;**104**(2):108-114

[18] Voulliaume D, Mojallal A, Comparin JP, Foyatier JL. Brûlures graves de la main et lambeaux: choix thérapeutiques et revue de la littérature. Annales de Chirurgie Plastique Esthétique. 2005;**50**(4):314-319

[19] DeBono R. A histological analysis of a high voltage electric current injury to an upper limb. Burns. 1999;**25**(6):541-547

[20] Karimi H, Momeni M, Vasigh M. Long term outcome and follow up of electrical injury. Journal of Acute Disease. 2015;**4**(2):107-111

[21] Mashreky SR, Hossain MJ, Rahman A, Biswas A, Khan TF, Rahman F. Epidemiology of electrical injury: Findings from a community based national survey in Bangladesh. Injury. 2012;**43**(1):113-116

[22] Maghsoudi H, Adyani Y, Ahmadian N. Electrical and lightning injuries. Journal of Burn Care & Research. 2007;**28**(2):255-261

[23] Carloni R, Pechevy L, Quignon R, Yassine A-H, Forme N, Zakine G. Electrical flash burns, about 33 cases. A 10-year retrospective study. Epidemiology, treatment and prevention. Annales de Chirurgie Plastique et Esthétique. 2015;**60**(2):123-130

[24] Dega S, Gnaneswar SG, Rao PR, Ramani P, Krishna DM. Electrical burn injuries. Burns. 2007;**33**(5):653-665

[25] Akçan R, Hilal A, Gülmen M, Çekin N. Childhood deaths due to electrocution in Adana, Turkey. Acta Paediatrica. 2007;**96**(3):443-445

[26] Bargues L, Leclerc T, Donat N, Jault P. Conséquences systémiques des brûlures étendues. Réanimation. 2009;**18**(8):687-693

[27] Pannucci CJ, Osborne NH, Jaber RM, Cederna PS, Wahl WL. Early fasciotomy in electrically injured patients as a marker for injury severity and deep venous thrombosis risk: An analysis of the national burn repository. Journal of Burn Care & Research. 2010;**31**(6):882-887

[28] Sahin I, Ozturk S, Alhan D, Açikel C, Isik S. Cost analysis of acute burn patients treated in a burn centre: The gulhane experience. Annals of Burns and Fire Disasters. 2011;**24**(1):9-13

[29] Tarim A, Ezer A. Electrical burn is still a major risk factor for amputations. Burns. 2013;**39**(2):354-357

[30] Chaouat M, Zakine G, Mimoun M. Principes de la prise en charge locale: Traitements chirurgicaux. Pathologie et Biologie. 2011;**59**(3):e57-e61

[31] Duhamel P, Rem K, Hounkpevi M, Brachet M, Duhoux A, Giraud O, et al. La chirurgie aiguë des brûlés: Etat actuel, voies de recherche et perspectives médecine et armées. 2015;**43**(2):165-174

[32] Lakhel A, Pradier J-P, Brachet M, Duhoux A, Duhamel P, Fossat S, et al. Chirurgie des brûlures graves au stade aigu. EMC–Techniques chirurgicales–Chirurgie plastique reconstructrice et esthétique. 2008;**3**(3):1-36

[33] Sauerbier M, Ofer N, Germann G, Baumeister S. Microvascular reconstruction in burn and electrical burn injuries of the severely traumatized upper extremity. Plastic and Reconstructive Surgery. 2007;**119**(2):605-615

[34] Ofer N, Baumeister S, Megerle K, Germann G, Sauerbier M. Current concepts of microvascular reconstruction for limb salvage in electrical burn injuries. Journal of Plastic, Reconstructive & Aesthetic Surgery. 2007;**60**(7):724-730

[35] Georgescu AV, Matei I, Ardelean F, Capota I. Microsurgical nonmicrovascular flaps in forearm and hand reconstruction. Microsurgery. 2007;**27**(5):384-394

[36] Chong SJ, Liang WH, Tan B-K. Use of multiple VAC devices in the management of extensive burns: The total body wrap concept. Burns. 2010;**36**(7):e127-e129

[37] Fette A. Children and their burned limbs. Burns. 2007;**33**(1):S20

[38] Hakkarainen AJ, Kukko H, Vuola J. Vacuum-assisted closure in deep extremity burns. Burns. 2009;**35**:S23-S24

[39] Ghavami Y, Mobayen MR, Vaghardoost R. Electrical burn injury: A five-year survey of 682 patients. Trauma Monthly. 2014;**19**(4). Available from: http://www.traumamon.com/?page=article&article_id=18748

[40] Piotrowski A, Fillet A-M, Perez P, Walkowiak P, Simon D, Corniere M-J, et al. Outcome of occupational electrical injuries among French electric company workers: A retrospective report of 311 cases, 1996-2005. Burns. 2014;**40**(3):480-488

[41] Chudasama S, Goverman J, Donaldson JH, van Aalst J, Cairns BA, Hultman CS. Does voltage predict return to work and neuropsychiatric sequelae following electrical burn injury? Annals of Plastic Surgery. 2010;**64**(5):522-525

[42] Tamam Y, Tamam C, Tamam B, Ustundag M, Orak M, Tasdemir N. Peripheral neuropathy after burn injury. European Review for Medical and Pharmacological Sciences. 2013;**17**(Suppl 1):107-111

[43] Bailey B, Gaudreault P, Thivierge RL. Neurologic and neuropsychological symptoms during the first year after an electric shock: Results of a prospective multicenter study. The American Journal of Emergency Medicine. 2008;**26**(4):413-418

[44] Cochran AJ, Essner R, Rose DM, Glass EC. Principles of sentinel lymph node identification: Background and clinical implications. Langenbeck's Archives of Surgery. 2000;**385**(4):252-260

[45] Ramati A, Rubin LH, Wicklund A, Pliskin NH, Ammar AN, Fink JW, et al. Psychiatric morbidity following electrical injury and its effects on cognitive functioning. General Hospital Psychiatry. 2009;**31**(4):360-366

Section 4

Scars: Post Surgery

Chapter 4

Endometriosis of Postoperative Scar

Andrei Plotski

Abstract

Endometriosis is seen in women during their reproductive age, where functional endometrial glands of the uterus and stromal component are observed outside the uterine cavity. Endometriosis in an operative scar is a rare event following mainly obstetric and gynecologic operation. Typical signs of scar endometriosis are cyclic pain and swelling tumor in the scar after obstetric or gynecologic operations. We present 24 cases of scar endometriosis with discussion and emphasis on variants of clinical signs, differential diagnostic, methods of treatment, and prevention.

Keywords: endometriosis, scar, laparotomy, incision, cesarean section

1. Introduction

Endometriosis is one of the most common diseases of the female genital tract. This pathology is characterized by the presence of the endometrial tissue outside the place of its usual localization. Commonly, in gynecological practice, we have to face pelvic endometriosis; however, extragenital endometriosis is described in different organs and body systems, including the intestines, urinary tract, thorax, umbilicus, etc. It is very difficult to establish the real frequency of extragenital endometriosis [1]. This is due to different approaches to accounting of the disease, treatment of patients in a variety of clinics, and underestimating of non-severe clinical signs. Among locations of endometriosis in the urinary tract, the lesion of the bladder is dominant, and in the gastrointestinal tract, lesions of the rectum and sigmoid colon [1]. Affection of the lungs occurs significantly rare. Endometriosis in a postoperative scar is a secondary process in scars after surgical procedures affecting the endometrium: cesarean section, hysterectomy, amniocentesis, etc. Nevertheless scar endometriosis occurs also after general surgery—appendectomy, cholecystectomy, and correction of hernias [2]. The term "endometrioma" is used for well-marked tumor-like lesions [3]. However, there may be a situation characterized by a typical clinic of endometriosis in the absence of a clearly defined lesion, and this makes diagnosis difficult. Its clinical diagnosis is confused with abscess, hematoma, suture granuloma, desmoid tumor, sarcoma, etc. Incidence rates for endometrioma associated with cesarean section have been reported to be 0.01–4% [3]. The incidence of endometrioma in episiotomy scars is much less than in abdominal wall scars. In this study we present 24 cases of endometriomas appearing after cesarean section, laparoscopic cystectomy, and perineal incision.

 IntechOpen

2. Case reports and discussion

We present 24 cases of scar endometriosis that we observed since 2003 till 2018. Mean age of patients was 29 years, in the range of 25–33.5 years. Twenty-two patients have previously undergone cesarean section, five of them were operated twice. Cesarean section was performed 5 (range 4–7) years ago. Clinical signs appeared during 1–3 years after the last cesarean section. More than half of the patients initially seek care from general surgeons and only after the examination were sent to a gynecologist. One patient suffers from endometriosis of postoperative scar after perineorrhaphy performed 23 years ago, and the last patient presents lesion in the region of left lateral trocar tract after removal of endometrioid ovarian cyst 6 months ago. It is interesting that 12 patients believed that the cause of their suffering was a non-gynecological disease, so they initially claimed to a general surgeon.

All patients after previous cesarean section presented painful tumor of a scar; palpable sizes of lesion were 45 (range 35–55) mm. Sometimes the lesion rises above the skin, but usually it is palpable deep in the tissue. The degree of pain increased during menses, and tumors became more swollen at that time—but only in 50% cases. Another 50% of patients suffered only from the presence of swelling in the area of the postoperative scar with moderate pain that was not associated with the menstrual cycle. One patient presented fistula in the angle of a scar with dark brown discharges during menstruation (**Figure 1**).

Endometriosis in the region of the perineum developed in a patient after childbirth for 14 years. She obtained medical care only after a slowly increasing lesion began to cause discomfort during sexual activity and walking. It was an unmovable swelling, 5–4–4 cm in sizes, almost woody in consistency. The moderate pain syndrome was not of a cyclical nature. Initially we suspected the pathology of Bartholin's gland, but later we were inclined to think about postoperative scar endometriosis. It should be noted that none of the patients examined by us had a history of genital endometriosis, although according to the literature this may be one in every fourth case [1].

All patients have undergone physical examination with obligatory ultrasound of postoperative scar for visualization of endometrioma (**Figure 2**). On ultrasound examination in all cases, we revealed hypoechoic nodules with irregular borders (**Figure 3**). Palpable tumors may have oval or irregular shape with or without clear marked boundaries. Internal structure was homogeneous only in one case; in others, tumors demonstrated different combinations of low echogenicity, hyperechoic

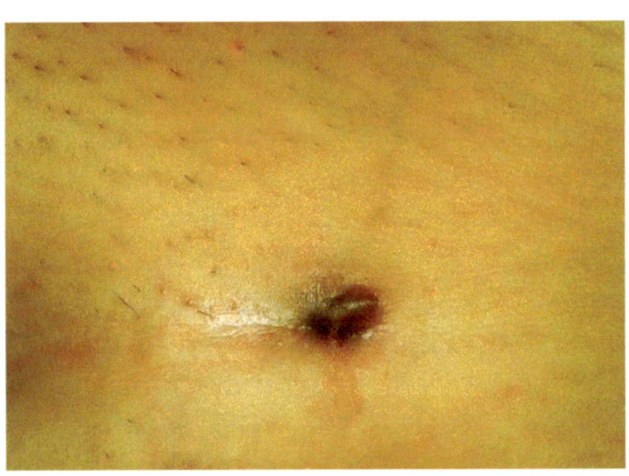

Figure 1.
Cutaneous endometrioid fistula.

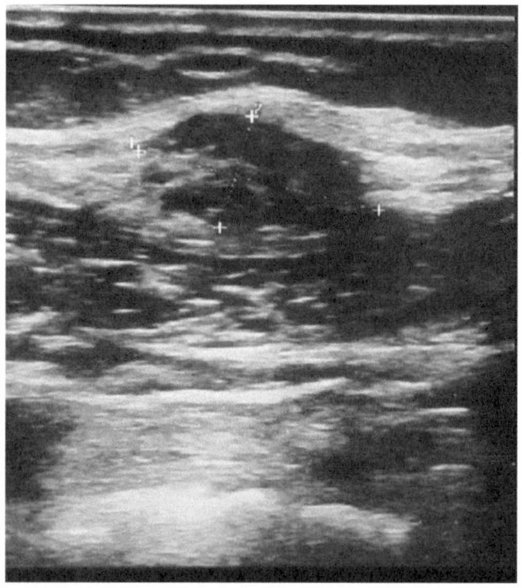

Figure 2.
Ultrasound image of endometrioma.

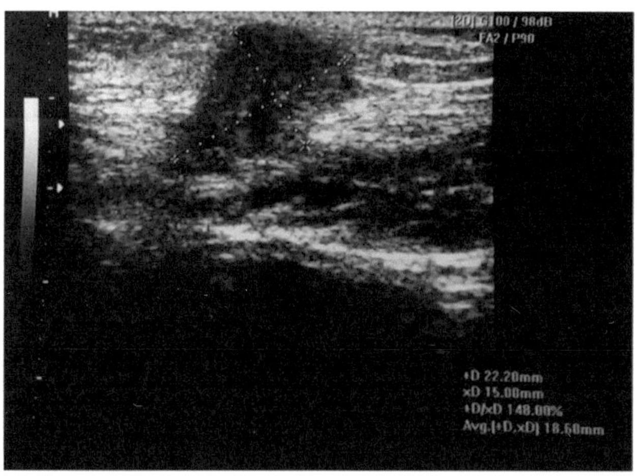

Figure 3.
Irregular borders of endometrioma.

inclusions, and anechoic cavities. All lesions were determined by good vascularization. It should be noted that in almost all cases the size of the structures on ultrasound was significantly less than palpable. It can be explained by the presence of perifocal inflammation.

All patients have undergone excision of tumors under general anesthesia with subsequent histological examination of the removed tissues (**Figure 4**). In 19 cases lesions were bordered by aponeurosis, muscles were intact, and wounds were sutured in layers.

Macroscopically excised structures usually were presented as a dense-consistency tissue with well-marked brown spots after incision (**Figure 5**) or without it (**Figure 6**). In three cases after operation, seroma with subfebrile temperature was formed; it was treated with antibiotics, aspiration drainage, and compressive bandage. Lesions were healed by secondary intension.

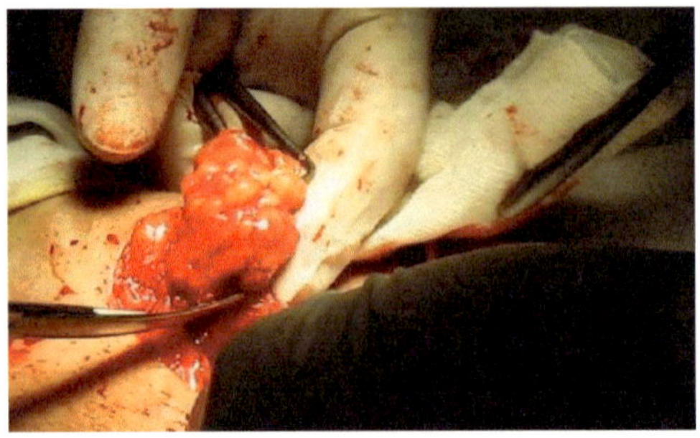

Figure 4.
Removal of endometrioma.

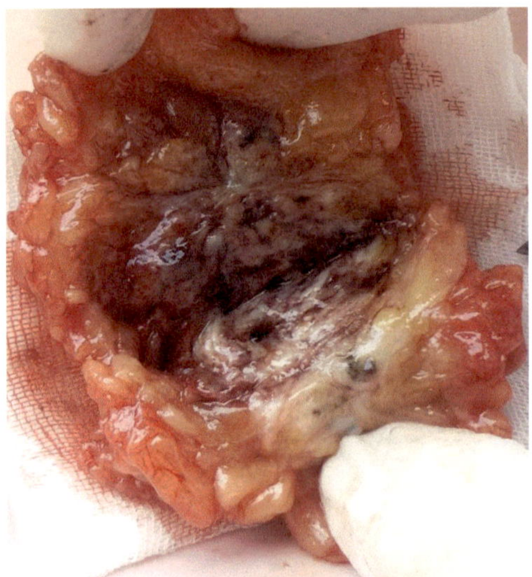

Figure 5.
Endometrioma after incision with brown spots.

The last three cases were not ordinary because lesions extended down to the subperitoneal layer and even to the peritoneal cavity. Localization of tumor in subperitoneal space was confirmed by MRI because the palpation data and the ultrasound results were doubtful in spite of typical "endometrioid" complains (**Figure 7**).

The patient suffered also from bilateral ovarian cysts (not endometrioid!) and has undergone laparoscopic cystectomy. And during the operation, we could visualize an endometrioid tumor located subperitoneally (**Figure 8**).

In two cases we have to perform laparotomy after excision of endometrioid lesion due to its spread to the abdominal cavity. In the first case, we removed tumor, observed pelvic cavity, found no signs of pelvic endometriosis, and repaired surgical wound. In the second case, tumor also spread to the abdominal cavity and connected with the low segment of the uterus. During excision we diagnosed injury of the posterior wall of the urinary bladder. The trauma of the urinary bladder was sutured by a urologist, Foley's catheter was inserted for 8 days, and wound was repaired. In this case we also revealed no evidence of pelvic endometriosis [4].

Excision of mass after perineorrhaphy was technically difficult due to woody consistency and severe adhesions with surrounding tissues.

Histological examination of the removed tissues revealed the presence of endometriosis in all cases except one. Endometrial tissue was in various proportions

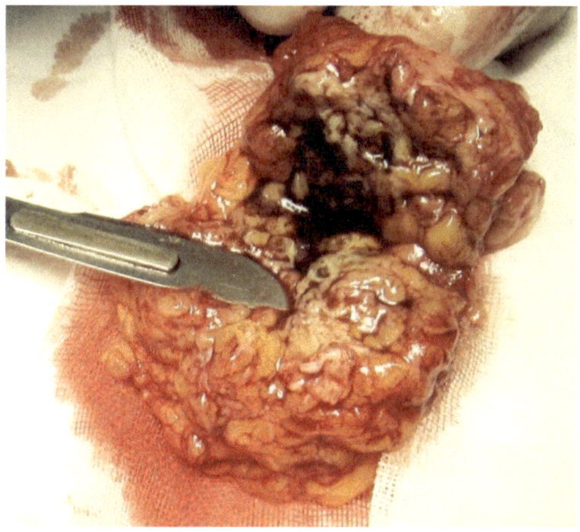

Figure 6.
Chocolate endometrioma.

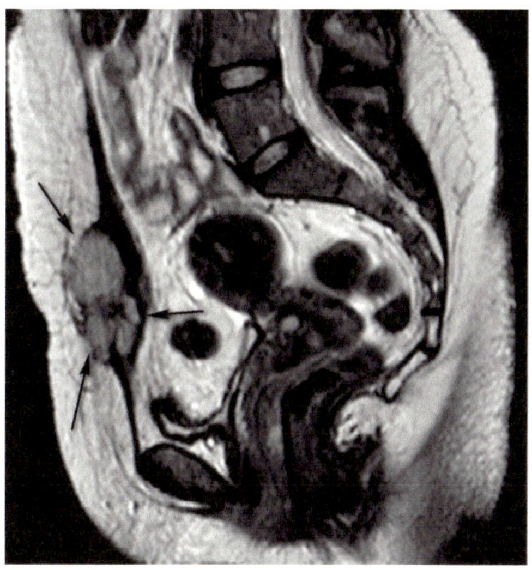

Figure 7.
MRI scan of endometrioma (black arrows).

with fibrous and fat tissues, even with suppuration of endometrial structures (after excision of lesion in the perineal region).

In all the cases, no recurrence was detected during the follow-up (1–12 years) except one—but it should not be considered as a recurrence, as the lesion appeared on the other side of the postoperative scar.

The final case was more interesting. As mentioned before, a 50-year-old patient was operated 6 months ago—bilateral adnexectomy by laparoscopic approach was performed due to endometrioid ovary cysts from both sides. Five months later the patient found the swelling painful mass in the region of the left trocar tract. Pain gradually increased, and slight redness of the skin appeared above the palpable tumor (**Figure 9**).

Adenocarcinoma was defined by histological examination after excision of tumor. We suppose that adenocarcinoma probably took place at the moment of the first laparoscopic operation in some parts of a cyst but was not revealed, so it was possible to develop into malignant tumor in trocar wound (we found out that the

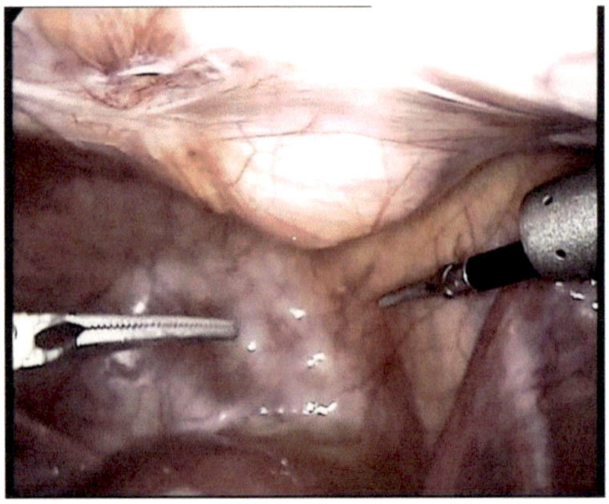

Figure 8.
Laparoscopic view of subperitoneal endometrioma.

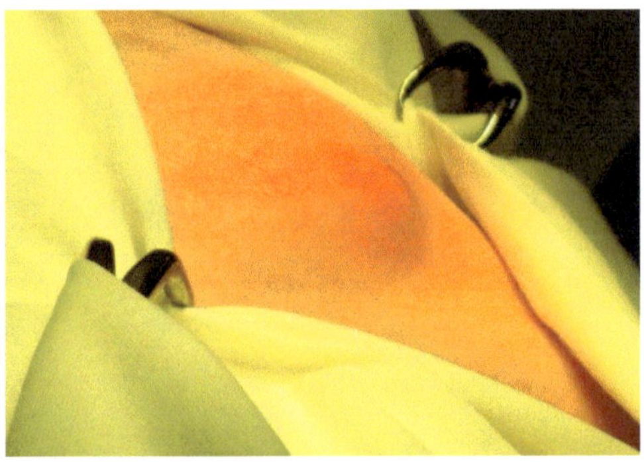

Figure 9.
View of "endometrioma" in the region of the trocar tract.

extraction of a cyst from the abdominal cavity was performed without using special containers). From the other side, it is difficult to exclude endometrial transformation in a malignant tumor [5]. Later the patient underwent several courses of chemotherapy.

Some theories have been put forward to explain the pathogenesis of endometriosis, such as lymphatic or hematogenous dissemination, coelomic metaplasia, and cell immunity change theory. The most prominent theory is that reflux of endometrial cells through the tubes into the peritoneal cavity during menstruation leads to pelvic endometriosis [2]. The viability and growth potential of desquamated menstrual endometrium have been demonstrated [6]. The metaplasia theory states that endometrioma arises due to metaplasia of pluripotential mesenchymal cells [3]. The transport theory suggests that endometrial cells may be transported to distant location, forming endometriomas during surgical procedures. The cause of surgical scar endometriosis is believed to be iatrogenic transplantation of the endometrium to the surgical wound. Evolution of knowledge about scar endometriosis is rather interesting. Review of the early literature shows a high association of abdominal scar endometriosis with a previous ventrofixation operation [7]. Then the operation of hysterotomy for termination of early pregnancy has been increasingly associated with this condition [6], and it was shown that early pregnancy endometrium was easier to transplant than the term pregnancy endometrium. In our study, one patient also was after termination of pregnancy by cesarean section at 18 weeks due to severe portal hypertension. In recent years, both genetic predisposition to endometriosis and the role of epigenetic factors are also actively discussed [8].

Nowadays, increasing of cesarean delivery—the main reason of abdominal scar endometriosis. Anyway, any operation on the uterus—it does not matter either ventrofixation or cesarean section—may lead to scar endometriosis due to the phenomenal viability of the endometrium [6, 7].

Endometriosis of postoperative scar can develop both after surgery performed by laparotomic approach and after laparoscopy in the area of the trocar opening, as well as in the perineal region after its incision during childbirth. Regardless of the type of intervention, the crucial point is that the endometrium implants on the wound surface and develops after it. Therefore, postoperative scar endometriosis is an example of iatrogenic endometrial transplantation to the wound surface. It is the transplantation theory which explains the appearance of the endometrium in the area of postoperative scar after non-gynecological operations—appendectomy, cholecystectomy, etc. In these cases, the operation is performed either during or immediately after menstruation, when the presence of the endometrium in the abdominal cavity is possibly as a result of reflux of endometrial cells through the fallopian tubes.

Despite the ectopic location, endometrial tissue is able to respond to hormonal effects, thereby causing clinical signs of disease. Endometriosis of postoperative scar is a typical example of extragenital endometriosis. But endometriosis of the postoperative scar is not only damage to the skin. In this situation, it is necessary to discuss the lesion of all tissues that were affected during surgical interventions.

The most common presenting symptom of endometrioma in a scar is a palpable mass associated with cyclic pain and swelling during menses [2]. Sometimes endometriomas may be multiple. Endometrial implants behave like normal endometrium in their response to hormones. Ovarian hormonal action on ectopic endometrial cells during menstrual period causes slight bleeding at the scar location with an inflammatory reaction and subsequent tissue repair. Thus, as each menstrual cycle goes by, the lesion increases in sizes, and this increasing might compromise the skin, subcutaneous cellular tissue, aponeurosis, and peritoneum. We observed these events in three of 19 cases. Also we consider that inflammatory changes of endometrial mass resulted in injuring the urinary bladder during excision.

If the symptoms are cyclic in the woman with a prior history of surgery on the uterus, then endometriosis should be the most likely consideration. It is practically pathognomonic. There is no need for advanced propaedeutics, and the diagnosis may be based on anamnesis and physical examination. Some authors describe a characteristic triad of periodic pain, tumor, and history of cesarean section [9]. When the patient complains are not cyclical, clinical diagnosis is impaired. Noncyclical symptoms are observed in 25–45% of patients with scar endometriosis. An association between scar endometriosis and pelvic endometriosis is possible to find in one quarter of the cases [9], but in our study we found none. The differential diagnosis of a mass in a scar includes keloid formation, suture granuloma (**Figure 10**), hematomas, abscess, desmoid tumor, postoperative hernia, lipoma, cyst, or even strange body.

It is also possible to face with a rare condition—the so-called gossipiboma. It is a foreign body-related inflammatory pseudotumor caused by retained non-resorbable or partially resorbable substances [10]. We observed a patient with cutaneous fistula, as casuistically it is possible to give an example of unusual clinical situation of a patient with an endometriotic uterocutaneous fistula. The patient presented a painful nodule on the cesarean scar, which was bleeding during menstruation.

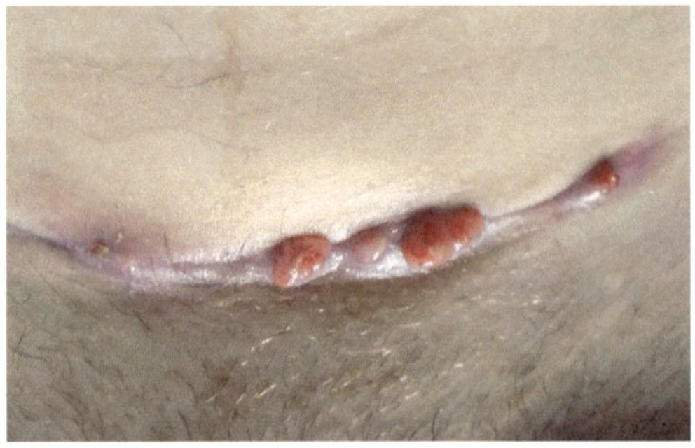

Figure 10.
Suture granuloma in 3 weeks after cesarean section.

It was established that the lesion extended to the uterine fundus, connecting the endometrial cavity with the skin [11].

Ultrasound examination and MRI may sometime aid in the diagnosis of scar mass, and fine needle aspiration cytology also has certain value in the diagnosis of scar endometriomas. The typical sonographic pattern is the presence of subcutaneous nodule, hypoechoic with hyperechoic strands and irregular margins. Sometime it is possible to visualize complete or incomplete hyperechoic ring around the nodule caused by a perifocal inflammatory reaction. In lesions larger than 3 cm, small cystic areas may be detected, possibly because of recent hemorrhage. In the typical case, a single peripheral vascular pedicle with arterial flow entering the nodule can be shown by color Doppler investigation. In very small lesions, this sign may be absent [12]. Because of high resolution of MRI, this technique makes it possible to identify smaller lesions and distinguish signs of organized hemorrhages within endometriomas. Moreover, MRI has better performance than computed tomography scans in relation to outlining the subcutaneous, muscle, and aponeurotic tissue layers (**Figure** 7).

In some cases thin needle puncture guided by ultrasound with cytological analysis helps to confirm diagnosis. In our study five of 24 patients have undergone this procedure before incision. However, its use is still controversial because of the risk of causing new implants at the puncture sites or perforating a hollow organ in the case of unrevealed or incarcerated hernia that simulated endometrioma.

Anyway imaging modalities remain nonspecific and do not modify the plan of treatment—wide surgical excision. Therapy with oral contraceptives, progestins, medroxyprogesterone acetate, and gonadotropin-releasing hormone agonists has been tried with minimal effects [4, 8]. In some patients the effects can be relatively long-lasting, but complete, permanent regression of endometriosis is rare with medical therapy. In our study we observed a patient treated with levonorgestrel-releasing intrauterine device during 1.5 years. Clinical signs of endometriosis disappeared, but lesion in the region of postoperative scar remained. After excision of this tumor, we found no typical "chocolate" inside (**Figure 11**).

Histological examination revealed "hollow" glands without epithelial cells. Treatment of this patient resulted in inhibition of endometrial tissue, but stromal component of endometriosis remained.

That is why for endometriosis of postoperative scar, total surgical excision is considered to be gold standard for both diagnosis and treatment. Resection must be complete with clear margins to prevent recurrence. The excision may be technically difficult depending on the depth and the size of mass. It is possible to use coagulation; it leads to smaller bleeding from infiltrated surrounded tissues. Sometimes

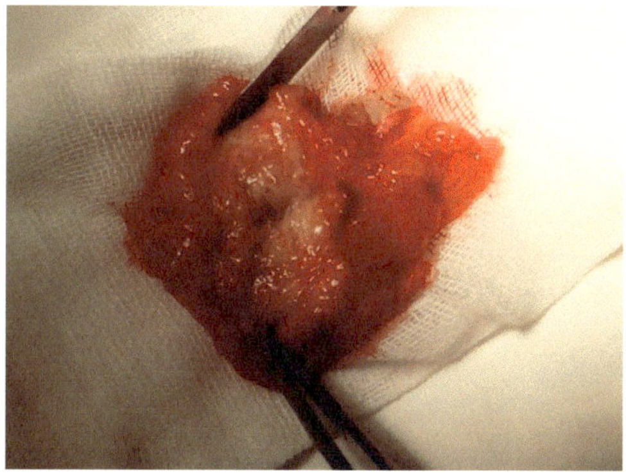

Figure 11.
Endometrioma after treatment with levonorgestrel-releasing system.

large defects in aponeurosis after excision require polypropylene mesh for repairing. Surgery should be performed some days before the menstrual period in order to avoid an inflammatory reaction and make tissue removal easier.

Scar endometriosis as well as endometriosis at other sites can become malignant. It is a rare event occurring in 0.3–1% of scar endometriomas. The phenomenon of malignancy arising in association with endometriosis was first described in 1925. Clear cell carcinoma is the most common histological subtype [5]. Frequent recurrence might indicate malignant degeneration of tumor. That is why longtime clinical follow-up is strongly recommended because malignant transformation might vary from a few months to more than 40 years.

In order to prevent scar endometriosis, some measures have been proposed. First of all, it is reasonable to close the peritoneal and visceral peritoneum with sutures at the time of cesarean section and perform an introflexed suture of the uterine incision and parietal peritoneum. Refusing these measures may increase the postoperative occurrence of an endometrioma in the scar. Second, it is not recommended to elevate the uterus out of the abdominal cavity during cesarean section or hysterotomy. Also it is recommended not to use the same instruments for hysterorrhaphy and suturing abdominal wall layers. At last, at the end of the surgery, the abdominal wall wound should be cleaned thoroughly and irrigated with high solution before closure. No measures of prevention have proven its efficiency, and all these measures were suggested without any evident scientific corroboration.

3. Conclusions

Twenty-four cases of endometriosis of postoperative scar have been presented. The occurrence of this type of extrapelvic endometriosis is supported by the iatrogenic implantation theory. Cyclic pain and swelling tumor in the scar after obstetric or gynecologic operation are typical signs of scar endometriosis. The absence of cyclic pain syndrome in the presence of a lesion in the region of the scar requires a differential diagnosis. Wide excision of tumor is the best way for treatment and final diagnosis.

Conflict of interest

The author declares no conflict of interest.

Author details

Andrei Plotski
Grodno State Medical University, Grodno, Belarus

*Address all correspondence to: androm1972@tut.by

References

[1] Hilaris GE, Payne CK, Osias J, Cannon W, Nezhat CR. Synchronous rectovaginal, urinary bladder, and pulmonary endometriosis. Journal of the Society of Laparoendoscopic Surgeons. 2005;**9**:78-82

[2] Akbulut S, Sevinc MM, Bakir S, Cakabay B, Sezgin A. Scar endometriosis in the abdominal wall: A predictable condition for experienced surgeons. Acta Chirurgica Belgica. 2010;**110**(3):303-307

[3] Kocher M, Hardie A, Schaefer A, McLaren T, Kovacs M. Cesarean-section scar endometrioma: A case report and review of the literature. Journal of Radiology Case Reports. 2017;**11**(12):16-26

[4] Plotski A, Garelik T, Mshar I, Parfenenko I, Garelic D. Endometriosis of postoperative scar: A report of five cases and short review of literature. Archives of Perinatal Medicine. 2013;**19**(4):229-232

[5] Ferrandina G, Paluzzi E, Fanfani F, Gentileschi S, Valentini AL, Mattoli MV, et al. Endometriosis-associated clear cell carcinoma arising in caesarean section scar: A case report and review of the literature. World Journal of Surgical Oncology. 2016;**14**(1):300

[6] Chambers DC. Endometriosis of the abdominal surgical scar following hysterotomy. Journal of the National Medical Association. 1975;**67**(6):465-467

[7] Harvey LP. Endometriosis in an abdominal scar. Proceedings of the Royal Society of Medicine. 1970;**63**(1):53

[8] Guo SW. Epigenetics of endometriosis. Molecular Human Reproduction. 2009;**15**(10):587-607

[9] Leite GK, Carvalho LF, Korkes H, Guazzelli TF, Kenj G, Viana AT. Scar endometrioma following obstetric surgical incisions: Retrospective study on 33 cases and review of the literature. São Paulo Medical Journal. 2009;**127**(5):270-277

[10] Pole G, Thomas B. A pictorial review of the many faces of gossipiboma: Observations in 6 cases. Polish Journal of Radiology. 2017;**82**:418-421

[11] Dragoumis K, Mikos T, Zafrakas M, Assimakopoulos E, Stamatopoulos P, Bontis J. Endometriotic uterocutaneous fistula after cesarean section: A case report. Gynecologic and Obstetric Investigation. 2004;**57**(2):90-92

[12] Francica G. Reliable clinical and sonographic findings in the diagnosis of abdominal wall endometriosis near cesarean section scar. World Journal of Radiology. 2012;**4**(4):135-140

Section 5

Modern Concepts of Treating Scars

Chapter 5

Keloids and Hypertrophic Scars Can Now Be Treated Completely by Multimodal Therapy, Including Surgery, Followed by Radiation and Corticosteroid Tape/Plaster

Rei Ogawa

Abstract

Keloids and hypertrophic scars are fibroproliferative disorders of the skin. Research over the last decade has markedly improved our understanding of the pathogenesis of these scars, in particular, the fact that both disorders are caused by prolonged inflammation that prevents the orderly healing of injured or irritated skin. This protracted inflammatory response is due to genetic, systemic, and local risk factors. Genetic factors include single nucleotide polymorphisms, while systemic factors include hypertension, pregnancy-related and other hormones, and aberrant cytokine levels. An important local factor is the mechanical force (tension) on the scar. These observations have greatly aided the development of therapies for these once-intractable scars. As a result, these scars are now regarded as being completely treatable. At present, we believe that the following combination of three therapies most reliably achieves a complete cure: surgery followed by radiation and the prolonged daily use of corticosteroid tape/plaster.

Keywords: keloid, hypertrophic scar, scar, scar contracture, fibroproliferative disorder, fibrosis, surgery, radiotherapy, corticosteroid, tape, plaster

1. Introduction

While keloids and hypertrophic scars have some tumor-like properties, they are actually inflammatory conditions that drive the excessive proliferation of dermal fibroblasts and the aberrant accumulation of dermal matrix [1]. These fibroproliferative disorders of the skin are caused by abnormal healing of injured or irritated skin. Common causes of injury and irritation are trauma, burn, surgery, vaccination, skin piercing, acne, and herpes zoster. The risk of developing keloids and hypertrophic scars is particularly high if the wound is deep enough to damage the reticular layer of the dermis and if various genetic, systemic, and/or local risk factors that prolong the inflammatory stage of wound healing are present. The protracted inflammation accelerates angiogenesis and induces the excessive accumulation of collagen. As a result, red and elevated scars that have an unappealing appearance arise. These scars also associate with intermittent pain, persistent itching, and a sensation of contraction. Moreover, if the wounds are located on the joints or mobile regions, including the neck, the resulting scars can develop into scar contractures. Thus, the primary end-points of treatments for keloids and hypertrophic scars should be functional improvement and relief from pain and itch. Another important goal is the esthetic improvement.

2. Causes of keloids and hypertrophic scars

A number of genetic, systemic, and local factors that influence the characteristics and quantity of keloids and hypertrophic scars have been identified [2]. The genetic causes of pathological scar development include single nucleotide polymorphisms [3, 4]. Moreover, our study showed that one of these polymorphisms associates significantly with clinically severe keloids [4]. It has been suggested that keloids are more influenced by genetic background than hypertrophic scars. This notion remains to be tested. To test it, it will be necessary to have a critical biomarker that reliably distinguishes keloids from hypertrophic scars. One possibility is keloidal collagen: it seems that this histological feature is only present in lesions that bear other classical hallmarks of keloids, including growth over the edges of the original wound. However, identification of other, nonpathology, biomarkers would be highly useful for addressing questions about the differences between keloids and hypertrophic scars in terms of their etiology, growth characteristics, and treatment responses.

In terms of systemic factors, adolescence and pregnancy appear to associate with a higher risk of developing pathological scars [5, 6]. Our recent study also showed that hypertension associates with the development of severe keloids [7, 8]. I believe that while these factors are not primary causes of keloid and hypertrophic scars, they do worsen the inflammation in the scar tissue, thereby accelerating and increasing angiogenesis and matrix production.

Of the many factors that contribute to pathological scar development is local mechanical forces, I believe that they play a particularly important role [9–11]. Keloids commonly adopt distinct site-specific shapes, namely, the typical butterfly, crab's claw, and dumbbell shapes on the shoulder, anterior chest, and upper arm, respectively. These shapes reflect the region-specific distribution of skin tension that then tugs repetitively or constantly on the wounds/scars. Moreover, keloids are rare on the upper eyelid. This reflects the fact that eyelid skin is always relaxed regardless of whether the eyes are open or closed. An exception may be earlobe keloids: the contribution of mechanical factors to the development of these keloids may be minor. Instead, the most likely local cause of these keloids is the repeated attaching and detaching of the piercing, which repeatedly injures the skin and heightens the risk of infection. Both the skin tension and repeated injury/infection trigger inflammation and the downstream fibroproliferative events. In summary, while skin tension itself may not be a primary cause of keloids and hypertrophic scars, it is likely to be an important local risk factor that worsens and prolongs the inflammation that drives the formation and/or progression of these fibroproliferative scars.

3. Standard treatment of keloids and hypertrophic scars

These findings have markedly improved our understanding of the pathogenesis of keloids and hypertrophic scars, which in turn has promoted the development of highly effective treatments for these once-intractable scars. At present, I believe that the most reliable approach is a combination of three therapies, namely, surgery, followed by radiation, and prolonged daily use of steroid tape/plaster. The addition of radiation and steroid tape/plaster to surgery reflects the point made above, namely, that keloids and hypertrophic scars are inflammatory disorders, and not tumors. Consequently, anti-inflammatory treatments are most effective for these lesions. Indeed, as will be described below, steroid tapes/plasters/injections on their own work well to reduce the volume of accumulated collagen in keloids and hypertrophic scars, thereby causing their mass to shrink. However, steroid treatments take a long time to achieve mass reduction. Consequently, with large lesions, they are best performed after surgery that rapidly removes the lesion mass. Radiation on its own also has mass-reducing effects because it appears to suppress angiogenesis, and therefore dampens the influx of inflammatory cells and factors into the scar. These anti-inflammatory properties of steroid and radiation mean that their application after mass-reducing surgery (which by itself provokes inflammatory responses) will prevent the recurrence of excised keloids and hypertrophic scars.

Below, we will describe each of the three modalities separately. Thereafter, we will describe the three modalities when used in our combination therapeutic protocol.

3.1 Surgery

Since surgical treatment itself induces inflammation, surgery alone associates with high rates of keloid and hypertrophic scar recurrence. Worse, the recurrent scars are often much bigger than the original lesions. Thus, unless the scar is a minor hypertrophic scar, the decision to surgically remove a pathological scar should be made very carefully and postoperative radiation therapy should always be performed. However, if keloids and hypertrophic scars have infected areas, such as inclusion cysts, these should be removed surgically. Another key indication for surgery is keloids and hypertrophic scars that result in scar contracture of the joints or mobile areas such as the neck. In this case, the contractures should be released by a combination of subcutaneous/fascial tensile reduction sutures, z-plasties, and regional/local flap transfer.

The main objective of surgery for keloids and hypertrophic scars is not only mass reduction, but it is also to reduce the mechanical tension on the scar or the wound that is left after surgical removal of the scar. This is due to the important role of mechanical tension in the development and progression of keloids and hypertrophic scars. This is reflected by the fact that the most effective surgical method for releasing scar contractures is to use a regional or local flap, especially skin-pedicled local flaps: these flaps are particularly useful because they expand naturally after surgery and are therefore not prone to postsurgical contractures [12]. In contrast, skin grafts do not expand, which means that skin grafting tends to generate secondary contractures that result in circular pathological scars around the grafted skin.

3.2 Radiation

Interestingly, keloids respond very well to primary radiation therapy (i.e., radiation monotherapy). This reflects the fact that radiotherapy has a strong anti-inflammatory effect. Primary radiation therapy is suitable for older patients or patients with severe (huge) keloids (**Figure 1**). Since the total radiation dose in these cases is relatively high (e.g., 5 Gy administered once a week for 5 weeks by superficial brachytherapy), it is necessary to apply the radiation carefully to prevent secondary radiation carcinogenesis. However, the risks of primary radiation therapy should be weighed against its tremendous benefits; in particular, the fact that it immediately alleviates the subjective symptoms of keloids such as pain and itching. Moreover, over the following year, it causes the color and thickness of the scars to progressively normalize.

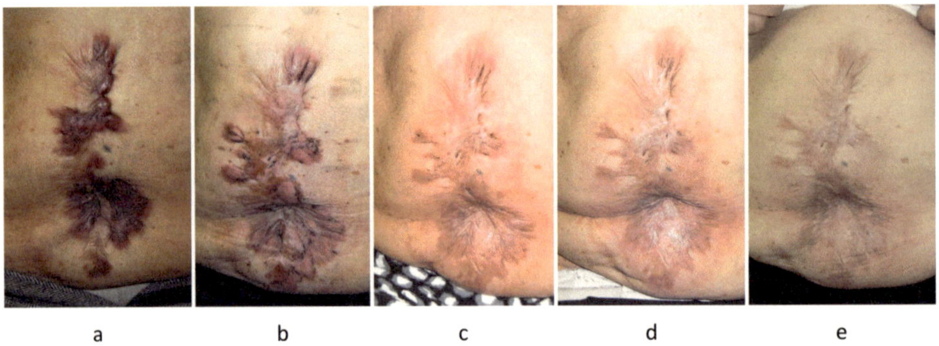

Figure 1.
A patient with severe abdominal keloids was effectively treated by radiation monotherapy. (a) View before treatment. (b) 4 months post-treatment. (c) 9 months post-treatment. (d) 14 months post-treatment. (e) 18 months post-treatment. A 68-year-old female was treated with high-dose-rate superficial brachytherapy. A total of 25 Gy was administered in five fractions over 5 days (i.e., 5 Gy was delivered once a week for 5 weeks). After 4 months of treatment, both the subjective and objective symptoms had improved dramatically. The keloids became mature scars 18 months after the treatment.

Radiation is also useful in the treatment of keloids and hypertrophic scars as a postsurgical modality [13–21]. As mentioned above, the main problem of surgery for pathological scars is recurrence. However, postsurgical radiation therapy can dramatically reduce these rates of recurrence. Use of the linear-quadratic model to calculate the biologically effective doses (BEDs) for various therapeutic radiation regimens after surgical excision of keloids showed that when the BED exceeds 30 Gy, the recurrence rate is less than 10%. Indeed, our review of the literature showed that to ensure maximum efficacy and safety, postoperative radiation for keloids in adults should involve the application of 10–20 Gy *via* daily fractions of 5 Gy.

Currently, we propose that the maximum dose of postoperative radiation therapy for surgically excised keloids is a BED of 30 Gy. A BED of 30 Gy can be obtained in several ways: a single fraction dose of 13 Gy, two fractions of 8 Gy, three fractions of 6 Gy, or four fractions of 5 Gy. In addition, recommended site-dependent dose protocols for the treatment of keloids are as follows: 18 Gy in three fractions over 3 days for the anterior chest wall, shoulder-scapular region, and suprapubic region; 8 Gy in a fraction over a day for the ear lobe; and 15 Gy in two fractions over 2 days for other sites.

It should be noted that the calculated BED of 30 Gy assumes that the α/β ratio for keloids is 10 (the α/β ratio is a measure of the radiosensitivity of a specific tissue). However, when Flickinger [21] investigated the α/β ratio of keloids, they found that it was as low as 2, which suggests that high doses with limited numbers of fractions is the best strategy to achieve low recurrence rates. At present, there is no widely accepted radiation regimen for keloid treatment. Further research on regimens that effectively prevent recurrence without elevating the risk of secondary carcinogenesis is welcome.

3.3 Corticosteroid tapes/plasters

Corticosteroid injections rapidly reduce the volume of a scar [22]. However, the downsides of corticosteroid injections include pain (caused by the injection itself) and difficulties associated with contraindications such as pregnancy, glaucoma, or Cushing's disease. This problem can be overcome by using steroid tapes/plasters. Most pediatric and older patients can be treated by steroid tapes/plaster alone because they have much thinner skin, which means that the steroids are easily absorbed (**Figure 2**). Corticosteroid tape/plasters on their own or in combination

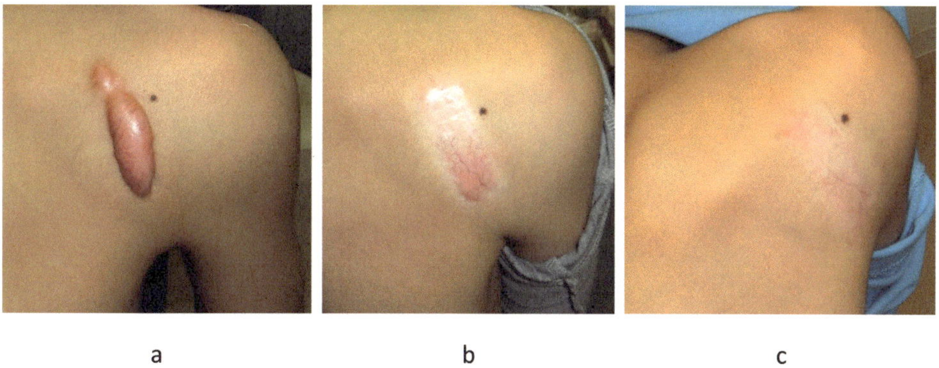

Figure 2.
A child with a mild keloid was effectively treated with steroid tape alone. (a) View before treatment. (b) After 16 months of treatment. (c) After 26 months of treatment. This 9-year-old boy had a mild right scapular keloid and was treated by fludroxycortide tape (Drenison® tape). The tape was placed on the keloid 24 h a day and was changed daily. The inflammation resolved completely. After 26 months of treatment, both the subjective and objective symptoms of the patient had improved dramatically (the case was cited from the article: Ogawa R, Akaishi S, Kuribayashi S, Miyashita T. Keloids and Hypertrophic Scars Can Now Be Cured Completely: Recent Progress in Our Understanding of the Pathogenesis of Keloids and Hypertrophic Scars and the Most Promising Current Therapeutic Strategy. J Nippon Med Sch. 2016;83(2):46–53).

with other therapies such as corticosteroid injection are also suitable for adults with minor keloids. Notably, postoperative application of corticosteroid tape/plasters significantly prevents the development of keloids and hypertrophic scars after surgery.

Steroid tape/plasters should be changed every day. Important tips regarding the treatment of keloids and hypertrophic scars with steroid tapes/plasters are as follows. First, the patient should continue to use the tapes/plasters until the elevated mass becomes flat and soft. Second, once the mass has become flat and soft, steroid tape/plaster use should be stopped, even if the scar is still red. This reflects the fact that if the patient continues to use the tape just because the scar is still red, capillarectasia will occur. This is because the steroid treatment thins the supporting structure of the blood vessels.

Steroid tape is available in the following three countries in slightly different preparations [22]. In the UK, the commercially available formulation comprises a fludroxycortide-impregnated tape (4 $\mu g/cm^2$). In the USA, a preparation containing 4 $\mu g/cm^2$ flurandrenolide (a medium-strength steroid) is available. In Japan, two steroid tape formulations are available, namely, a 4 $\mu g/cm^2$ fludroxycortide tape (medium-strength) and a 20 $\mu g/cm^2$ deprodone propionate tape (higher potency steroid). In our experience, deprodone propionate tape is the most effective tape for the treatment and prevention of keloids.

4. Combination treatment for severe keloids and hypertrophic scars

If a patient has severe keloids with infected areas or scar contractures, surgery should be performed (**Figure 3**). If the keloids are too large to be removed in their entirety, the surgeon can resect the region of contracture or infection. The resulting defects can then be covered by a regional/local flap. Surgery should also be performed if the keloid growth causes significant deformity and the keloid does not respond to nonsurgical therapies. An example of severely deforming earlobe keloids is shown in **Figure 4**. Such keloids can be treated by the core excision method, where the fibrous reticular layer of the keloid (i.e., the core of the earlobe keloid) is extirpated and the epidermis and papillary layer of the dermis is preserved as a thin flap.

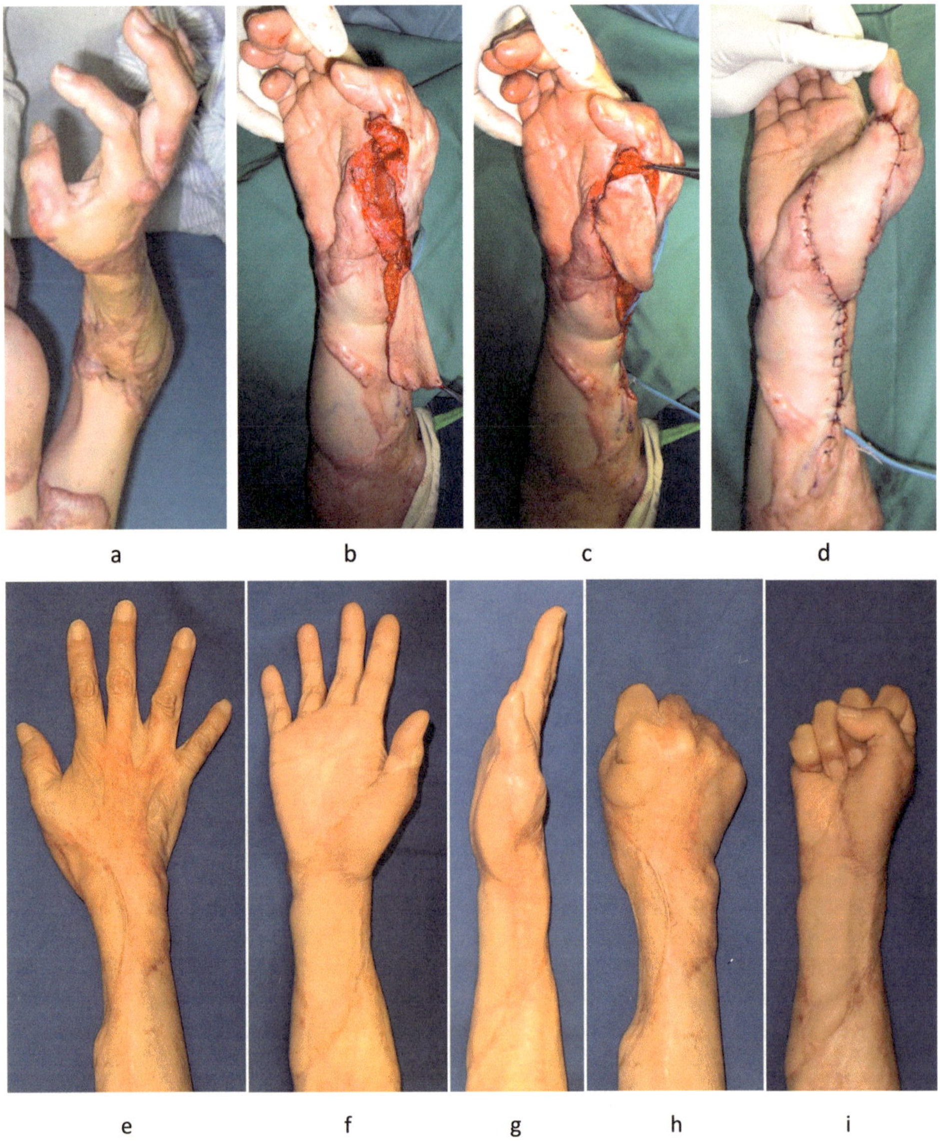

Figure 3.
A patient with an upper limb keloid was effectively treated by surgery and postoperative radiotherapy. (a) Preoperative view. (b) Removal of the hand and wrist keloids and harvest of the flap. (c) Flap rotation. (d) The recipient site immediately after surgery. (e–i) 5 years after the operation. This 63-year-old female had hypertension together with severe keloids of an unknown origin (folliculitis was suspected) that covered her right elbow, wrist joint, and thumb and made it difficult for her to use her right hand. The contractures were released by surgery with a distally based radial forearm flap followed by adjuvant 4-MeV electron beam irradiation therapy (15 Gy/three fractions for 3 days) (the case was cited from the article: Ogawa R, Arima J, Ono S, Hyakusoku H. CASE REPORT Total Management of a Severe Case of Systemic Keloids Associated With High Blood Pressure (Hypertension): Clinical Symptoms of Keloids May Be Aggravated by Hypertension. Eplasty. 2013 Jun 3;13:e25).

While these surgical approaches on their own associate with a relatively high risk of recurrence, this risk can be significantly reduced by combining surgery with postoperative radiotherapy and prolonged corticosteroid tape/plaster application. Thus, after the operation, both the donor and recipient sites of the flap should be irradiated to prevent the new formation of keloids. Notably, when partial resection or core extirpation is followed by postoperative radiotherapy, any remaining keloids around the flap (which do not undergo radiotherapy) also improve (**Figure 3**). This

DOI: http://dx.doi.org/10.5772/intechopen.84178

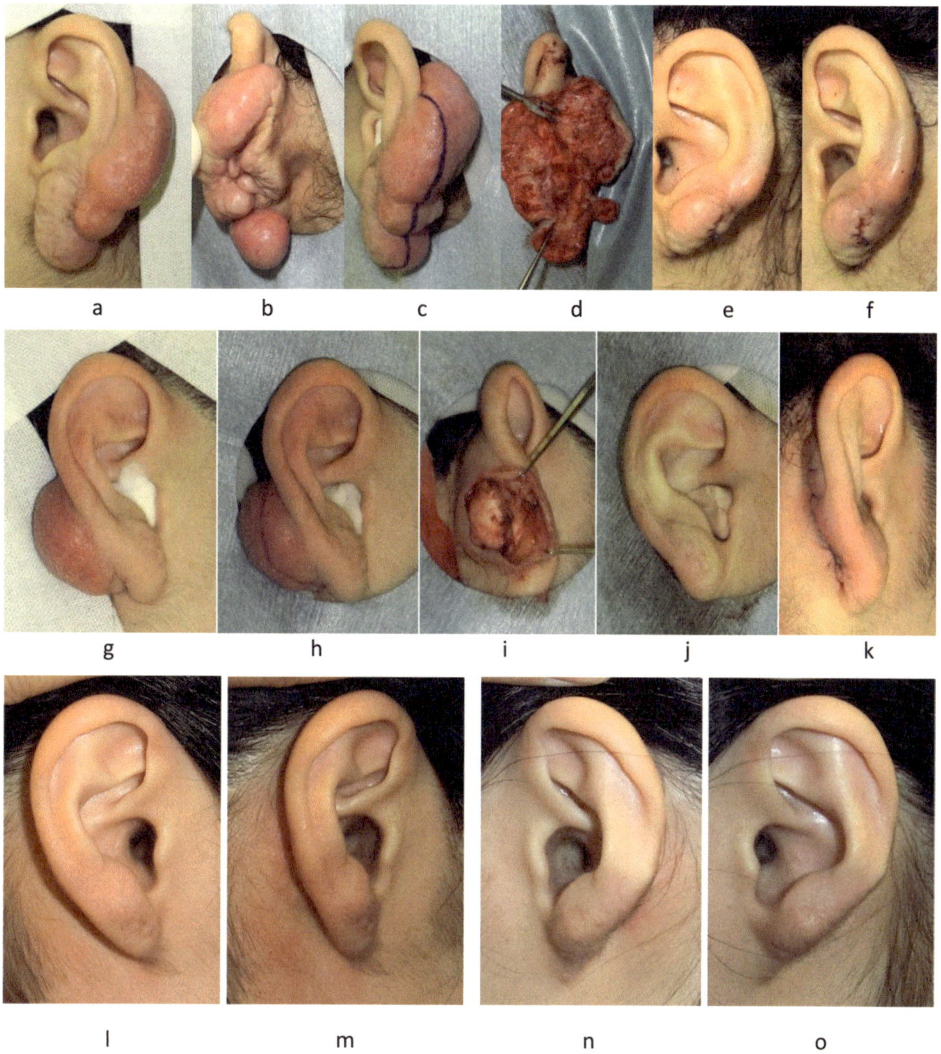

Figure 4.
A patient with bilateral ear keloids was effectively treated by surgery and postoperative radiotherapy. (a, b) Preoperative view of the left ear. (c) Design of the incision on the left ear. (d) Intraoperative view of the left ear. (e, f) The left ear immediately after surgery. (g) Preoperative view of the right ear. (h) Design of the incision on the right ear. (i) Intraoperative view (the right ear). (j, k) The right ear immediately after surgery. (l, m) The right ear 14 months after surgery. (n, o) The left ear 14 months after surgery. A 37-year-old Japanese woman with multiple keloids was diagnosed with multicentric type Castleman's disease. She was treated with systemic administration of steroid for Castleman's disease but the treatment did not improve her keloids. We removed both auricular keloids by using the core excision method. On postoperative days 1, 2, and 3, the patient received a total radiation dose of 15 Gy in three fractions over 3 days. The radiation was delivered by a 4 MeV electron beam. Histopathological examination of the resected tissues showed the absence of abnormal lymphocytes or plasma cell infiltration. Consequently, the auricular lesions were diagnosed definitively as keloids (the case was cited from the article: Quong WL, Kozai Y, Ogawa R. A Case of Keloids Complicated by Castleman's Disease: Interleukin-6 as a Keloid Risk Factor. Plast Reconstr Surg Glob Open. 2017 May 16;5(5):e1336).

reflects the fact that the flap releases tension, which in turn decreases the inflammation in the remnant keloids. The high risk of recurrence in these severe cases can be further reduced by the routine application of corticosteroid tape/plasters on the operated area that are changed daily. In general, we recommend patients to use tape/plasters for at least 6 months after the surgery and radiotherapy, or until the scar becomes soft. Long-term follow-up is necessary because if the scars start to stiffen again, corticosteroid tape/plasters should be re-applied. In general, it will

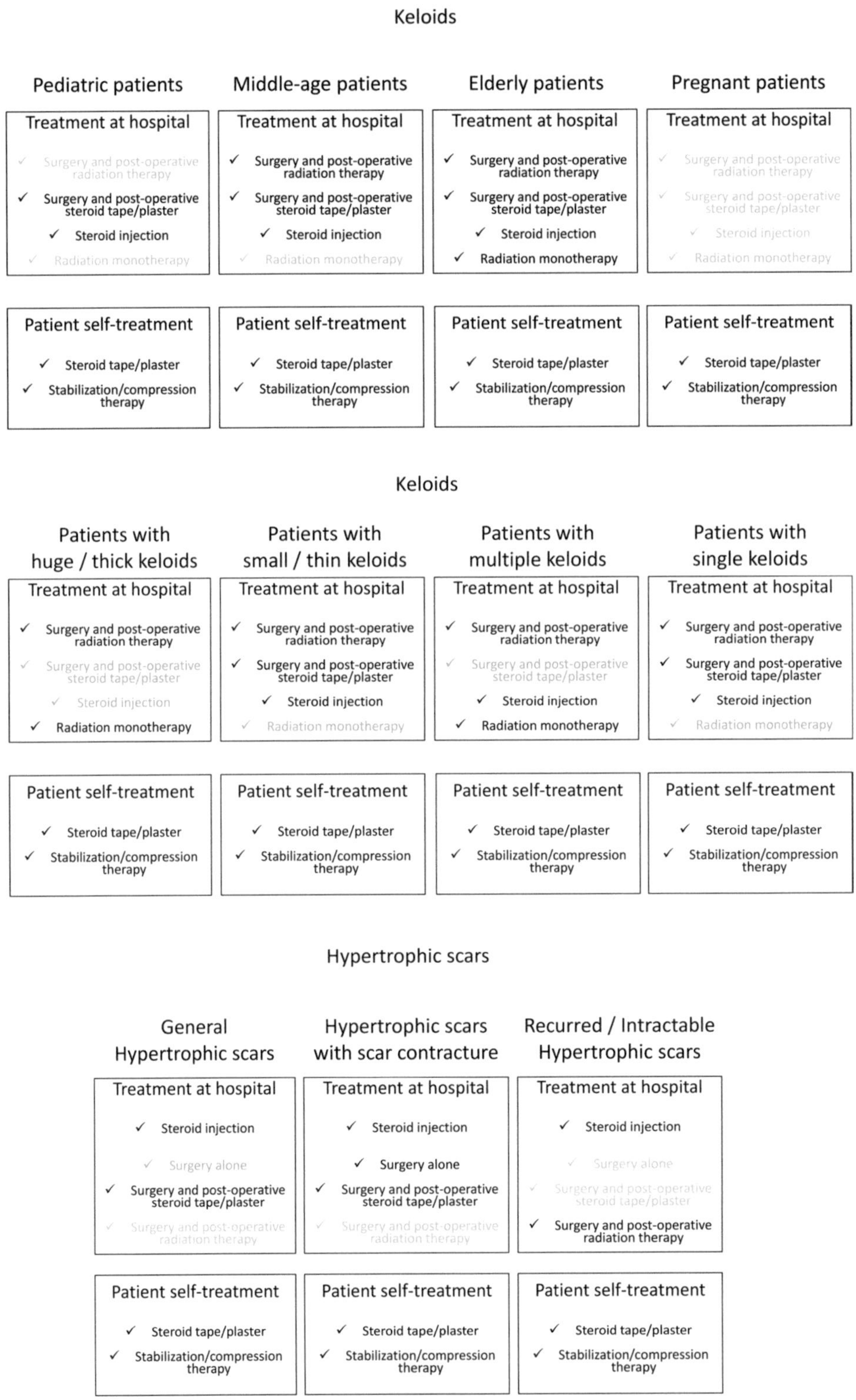

Figure 5.
Algorithm for selecting keloid and hypertrophic scar treatment modalities. Particular care should be taken when selecting the treatment for growing children and pregnant women with keloids and hypertrophic scars. In our facility, pediatric patients (<20 years of age) and pregnant women are not treated with radiation. Invasive surgery in pregnant women is also avoided. In these cases, the primary treatment choice should be steroid tape/plaster together with stabilization/compression therapy that reduces the tension on the scar.

take at least 2 years before combination therapy-treated keloids and hypertrophic scars mature. It is important to make clear to the patient before this therapy starts that the protocol has a long duration. Nevertheless, close monitoring and assiduous re-application of steroid tape/plasters have an excellent chance of converting postoperative keloid sites into mature scars.

It should be noted that our combination therapy is not suitable for growing children and pregnant women. In our facility, we do not treat pediatric patients (<20 years of age) or pregnant women with radiation. Moreover, invasive treatments such as surgery are not performed during pregnancy. The primary choice of treatment for children and pregnant women with keloids and hypertrophic scars should be steroid tape/plaster on its own (**Figure 5**).

Author details

Rei Ogawa
Department of Plastic, Reconstructive and Aesthetic Surgery, Nippon Medical School Hospital, Tokyo, Japan

*Address all correspondence to: r.ogawa@nms.ac.jp

References

[1] Ogawa R. Keloid and hypertrophic scars are the result of chronic inflammation in the reticular dermis. International Journal of Molecular Sciences. 2017;**18**(3):E606

[2] Huang C, Murphy GF, Akaishi S, Ogawa R. Keloids and hypertrophic scars: Update and future directions. Plastic and Reconstructive Surgery. Global Open. 2013;**1**(4):e25

[3] Nakashima M, Chung S, Takahashi A, Kamatani N, Kawaguchi T, Tsunoda T, et al. A genome-wide association study identifies four susceptibility loci for keloid in the Japanese population. Nature Genetics. 2010;**42**(9):768-771

[4] Ogawa R, Watanabe A, Than Naing B, Sasaki M, Fujita A, Akaishi S, et al. Associations between keloid severity and single-nucleotide polymorphisms: Importance of rs8032158 as a biomarker of keloid severity. The Journal of Investigative Dermatology. 2014;**134**(7):2041-2043

[5] Moustafa MF, Abdel-Fattah MA, Abdel-Fattah DC. Presumptive evidence of the effect of pregnancy estrogens on keloid growth. Case report. Plastic and Reconstructive Surgery. 1975;**56**(4):450-453

[6] Mendelsohn ME, Karas RH. Estrogen and the blood vessel wall. Current Opinion in Cardiology. 1994;**9**(5):619-626

[7] Arima J, Huang C, Rosner B, Akaishi S, Ogawa R. Hypertension: A systemic key to understanding local keloid severity. Wound Repair and Regeneration. 2015;**23**(2):213-221

[8] Huang C, Ogawa R. The link between hypertension and pathological scarring: Does hypertension cause or promote keloid and hypertrophic scar pathogenesis? Wound Repair and Regeneration. 2014;**22**(4):462-466

[9] Ogawa R, Okai K, Tokumura F, Mori K, Ohmori Y, Huang C, et al. The relationship between skin stretching/contraction and pathologic scarring: The important role of mechanical forces in keloid generation. Wound Repair and Regeneration. 2012;**20**(2):149-157

[10] Ogawa R, Akaishi S, Huang C, Dohi T, Aoki M, Omori Y, et al. Clinical applications of basic research that shows reducing skin tension could prevent and treat abnormal scarring: The importance of fascial/subcutaneous tensile reduction sutures and flap surgery for keloid and hypertrophic scar reconstruction. Journal of Nippon Medical School. 2011;**78**(2):68-76

[11] Akaishi S, Akimoto M, Ogawa R, Hyakusoku H. The relationship between keloid growth pattern and stretching tension: Visual analysis using the finite element method. Annals of Plastic Surgery. 2008;**60**(4):445-451

[12] Yoshino Y, Kubomura K, Ueda H, Tsuge T, Ogawa R. Extension of flaps associated with burn scar reconstruction: A key difference between island and skin-pedicled flaps. Burns. 2018;**44**(3):683-691

[13] Ogawa R. The most current algorithms for the treatment and prevention of hypertrophic scars and keloids. Plastic and Reconstructive Surgery. 2010;**125**(2):557-568

[14] Norris JE. Superficial x-ray therapy in keloid management: A retrospective study of 24 cases and literature review. Plastic and Reconstructive Surgery. 1995;**95**(6):1051-1055

[15] Enhamre A, Hammar H. Treatment of keloids with excision and postoperative X-ray irradiation. Dermatologica. 1983;**167**(2):90-93

[16] Guix B, Henríquez I, Andrés A, Finestres F, Tello JI, Martínez A.

Treatment of keloids by high-dose-rate brachytherapy: A seven-year study. International Journal of Radiation Oncology, Biology, Physics. 2001;**50**(1, 1): 167-172

[17] Kuribayashi S, Miyashita T, Ozawa Y, Iwano M, Ogawa R, Akaishi S, et al. Post-keloidectomy irradiation using high-dose-rate superficial brachytherapy. Journal of Radiation Research. 2011;**52**(3):365-368

[18] Ogawa R, Miyashita T, Hyakusoku H, Akaishi S, Kuribayashi S, Tateno A. Postoperative radiation protocol for keloids and hypertrophic scars: Statistical analysis of 370 sites followed for over 18 months. Annals of Plastic Surgery. 2007;**59**(6):688-691

[19] Ogawa R, Mitsuhashi K, Hyakusoku H, Miyashita T. Postoperative electron-beam irradiation therapy for keloids and hypertrophic scars: Retrospective study of 147 cases followed for more than 18 months. Plastic and Reconstructive Surgery. 2003;**111**(2):547-553

[20] Lo TC, Seckel BR, Salzman FA, Wright KA. Single-dose electron beam irradiation in treatment and prevention of keloids and hypertrophic scars. Radiotherapy and Oncology. 1990;**19**(3):267-272

[21] Flickinger JC. A radiobiological analysis of multicenter data for postoperative keloid radiotherapy. International Journal of Radiation Oncology, Biology, Physics. 2011;**79**(4):1164-1170

[22] Goutos I, Ogawa R. Steroid tape: A promising adjunct to scar management. Scars, Burns & Healing. 2017;**3**:2059513117690937

Chapter 6

Scars: A New Point of View in Plastic Surgery

Gustavo E. Prezzavento

Abstract

The issue of achieving esthetically pleasing surgical scars has gained prominence in recent years, with the emergence of the concept of the "imperceptible scar," which is expected by patients of not only cosmetic but also reconstructive surgery. Current research in reconstructive surgery focuses on obtaining high-quality results in the minimum number of steps, with a view to "doing it right the first time." However, there is no uniform approach to scar treatment, which is partly due to a lack of consensus regarding the most effective healing methods. This chapter aims at shedding new light to discussion by putting forward two different procedures that enhance scar results in cosmetic and reconstructive surgeries by applying a topical treatment with active ingredients and by combining cadaver and artificial skin as dermal substitutes, respectively. The effectiveness of these treatments is shown by means of objective, quantifiable data collected as a result of studies and postoperative follow-ups carried out at Hospital Alemán in Buenos Aires.

Keywords: scars, surgical wound, wound healing, reconstructive surgery, esthetic surgery

1. Introduction

Scars are a natural part of dermal healing following lacerations, incisions, or tissue loss. Wound healing, which is a natural process of tissue repair, consists of three phases: inflammation, fibroplasia, and maturation. The healing tissue generates changes in the cutaneous architecture, which renders the skin surrounding the scar different from the rest of the skin in terms of color, thickness, elasticity, texture, and degree of contraction [1]. In surgical procedures, scars, which are the only visible sequela of the intervention, result from the reparation process undergone by the skin to heal the wounds caused by surgery or trauma. Because of its impact in scarring, considerable importance is placed on the closure of a surgical incision, which is the final phase of the intervention [2]. The ideal scar is narrow, flat, level with surrounding tissue, and difficult for the untrained eye to see due to color match and placement parallel to relaxed skin tension lines. In contrast, hypertrophic, keloidal, dyspigmented, widened, contracted, or atrophic scars can be unsightly and/or cause functional limitations, which patients often perceive as a problem.

Thus, when the scar has unfavorable characteristics, scar revision is often indicated. Furthermore, as poor-quality healing of an incision can constitute a disabling pathology [3], scar treatment should not be considered as a trivial part of the intervention. On the contrary, wound treatment and care after surgery of any kind, including esthetic or reconstructive interventions, should be initiated early.

In order to arrive at an effective esthetic and functional outcome, surgeons must be familiar with the different scar treatments available, and they must also know how to prevent scars and how to reduce them after surgery. In this sense, it should be borne in mind that, while there exist multiple treatment modalities, none of them guarantees a 100% success rate. Current guidelines suggest a multimodal approach to treating scars but there is no gold standard for their treatment. In this chapter, we will present two new ways to treat scars following plastic surgery. As explained in the following sections, these techniques were successfully implemented in a number of cases, and their comparative advantages regarding other methods were also evaluated. We hope that our contribution will help point in the direction toward an effective, uniform standard.

The first part of our research deals with cosmetic surgery scars, which generally receive different topical treatments that help maintain the moisture and the plasticity of the wound. Besides, these treatments prevent wound contamination or infection, which would delay healing. We have analyzed and compared the results of two of these treatment options and found that the best functional and esthetic results are obtained when using a cream with active ingredients. The second part of our research revolves around the combined use of two skin substitutes, cadaver skin and artificial skin, so as to obtain improved results in reconstructive surgery after trauma injuries with abnormal wound healing in response to skin trauma or inflammation. Employing dermal substitutes result in a better regeneration of the dermis and in dermal fibroblast optimization. In the next sections, we will present a detailed account of the two studies we have carried out, which will allow us to further discuss the aforementioned techniques to optimize surgical scars.

2. Topical treatment of cosmetic surgery scars

As we have already mentioned, the first study involved the comparison and evaluation of two topical treatments applied to scars resulting from cosmetic surgery. One was a cream containing 1 g of silver sulfadiazine, 248,000 IU of vitamin A and 0.666 g of lidocaine in each 100 g of product (Platsul-A®, Soubeiran Chobet Laboratory, Autonomous City of Buenos Aires, Argentina) (cream A), and the other was a moisturizing cream based on petrolatum, keto-stearyl alcohol, glycerin, and water without any active ingredient (cream B). About 32 patients participated in the study; 24 with bilateral breast implants and 8 with face and neck lifts, hence totaling 64 scars. The study included patients of both sexes: 31 women and 1 man, with ages ranging from 22 to 64 years (mean of 41 years). All patients received both topical treatments under study, each of their postsurgical scars (right and left) being applied one of the creams at random. We monitored patients for 1 month after the beginning of treatment, meeting them at an initial appointment and at subsequent appointments after 3, 6, 9, 16, 23, and 30 days from the intervention. Each patient's progress was checked by the same medical examiner.

In these appointments, we measured the length and width of the scars to determine their total surface and assessed them in accordance with the Vancouver scar scale (VSS) and the patient and observer objective assessment scale (POSAS). We evaluated (1) the surface area of each scar by multiplying its length by its width, as measured with a ruler with graduation, (2) the quality of each scar as assessed by the VSS, [4] taking into account the parameters of pigmentation, vascularity, and thickness, and (3) the patient's perception of each scar as appraised by the POSAS, [5] by having them rank a series of symptomatic and esthetic parameters. The results are reported as follows, discriminated on the basis of the type of surgery performed.

2.1 Surface area of each scar

In the group of patients with breast implants, the percentage of change did not differ significantly between the two treatments studied in the appointments of days 3, 6, 9, 16, and 23. On day 30, however, we detected a statistically significant difference (P = 0.017). The percentage of decrease was significantly higher in the scars treated with the cream with silver sulfadiazine, vitamin A, and lidocaine (cream A) than in those treated with the cream without active ingredients (cream B) (18.6 and 9.5%, respectively) (**Table 1**). In the group of patients with face and neck lift, there was no significant difference between the percentage of change achieved due to the two treatments on days 3, 6, 9, and 16. Nevertheless, on days 23 and 30, we encountered a statistically significant difference (P = 0.026 and P = 0.007, respectively). The percentage of decrease was significantly higher in the scars treated with cream A than in those that had been treated with cream B. On day 23, the surface area of the scars treated with cream A had decreased, on average, by 14.8%, while that of the scars treated with cream B had increased, on average, by 24.9%. On day 30, the surface area of the scars treated with cream A had decreased, on average, by 19.1%, whereas that of the scars treated with cream B had increased, on average, by 22.2% (**Table 2**). **Figure 1** shows the changes in the surface area of each patient's scars on days 23 and 30 with respect to the initial appointment and classifies the results according to the type of surgery undergone and the treatment received. As we can see, more favorable results were obtained with cream A than with cream B, except in the case of two patients with breast implants (patients No. 7 and 12).

2.2 Vancouver scar scale

The VSS assigns values to the scar pigmentation, vascularity, and thickness, which are then added to obtain a total. Although the score may vary between 0 and 10, the average of the initial scores in our study was 2.7 and the maximum value observed throughout the study was 5. We conducted the analysis taking into account the absolute change in the VSS score with respect to the initiation of treatment (day 0). Results are expressed in absolute values. The analysis is carried out separately for each group of patients, depending on the type of surgery, on days 3, 6, 9, 16, 23, and 30.

In the breast implant patient group, the VSS score change did not differ significantly between treatments on days 3, 6, 9, and 16. On days 23 and 30, nonetheless,

Days	Average percentage of change of the surface area as from treatment onset (breast implant)		P
	Cream A (%)	Cream B (%)	
3	4.2	0.0	0.97 (NS)
9	2.6	3.7	0.37 (NS)
16	−1.8	−6.0	0.40 (NS)
23	−12.8	−7.2	0.089 (NS)
30	−18.6	−9.5	0.017*

NS: not significant. *Significant: at 5%.*

Table 1.
Average percentage of change of the surface area of the scars treated with silver sulfadiazine, vitamin A, and lidocaine (cream A) and with a cream without active ingredients (cream B) in patients with breast implants after 3, 6, 9, 16, 23, and 30 days from the onset of the topical treatment.

Days	Average percentage of change of the surface area as from treatment onset (face and neck lift)		P
	Cream A (%)	Cream B (%)	
3	12.5	12.5	+
6	12.5	12.5	+
9	12.3	12.4	0.60 (NS)
16	2.1	24.9	0.07 (NS)
23	−14.8	24.9	0.026*
30	−19.1	22.2	0.007**

NS: not significant.
**Significant at 5%.*
***Significant at 1%.*
+*No surface area changes were perceived in any patient in either of the treatments.*

Table 2.
Average percentage of change of the surface area of the scars treated with silver sulfadiazine, vitamin A, and lidocaine (cream A) and with a cream without active ingredients (cream B) in patients with face lift after 3, 6, 9, 16, 23, and 30 days from the onset of the topical treatment.

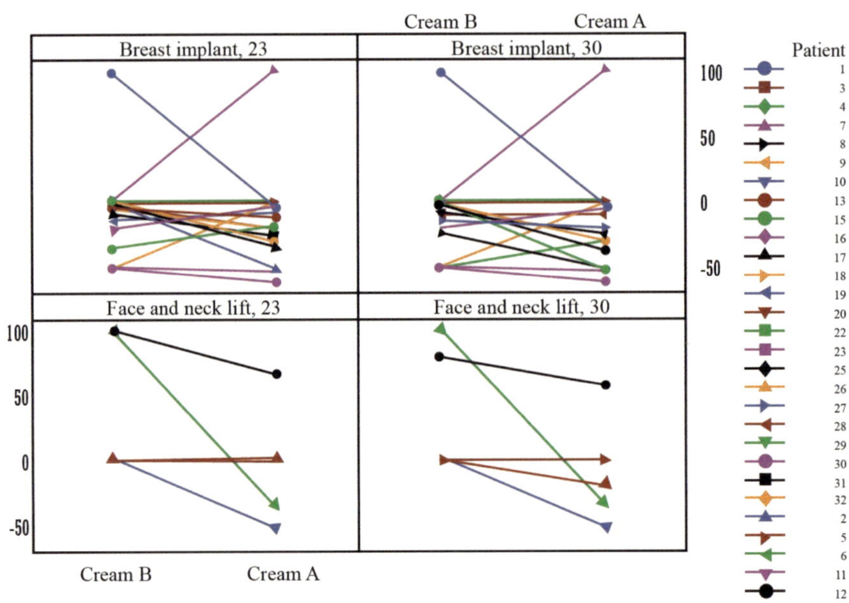

Figure 1.
Percentage changes of the scar surface area, per patient after 23 and 30 days from treatment onset.

we noticed a statistically significant difference (P = 0.02 and P = 0.006, respectively). The decrease was significantly higher in the scars treated with cream A in comparison with those treated with cream B. On day 23, the score of the scars treated with cream A decreased by 1.13 points average, while that of the scars treated with cream B increased by 0.04 points average. On day 30, the average score decrease was of 1.88 points in those treated with cream A and of 0.42 points in those treated with cream B (**Table 3**).

In the group of patients with face and neck lift, the change in the VSS score did not differ significantly between treatments after 3 days. Yet, in all of the following appointments, a statistically significant difference ($P < 0.05$) was observed. The reduction of the score was significantly higher in scars treated with cream A than in

Days	Average change in the VSS score as from treatment onset (breast implant)		P
	Cream A	Cream B	
3	0.33	0.21	0.80 (NS)
6	0.13	0.29	0.30 (NS)
9	−0.21	0.46	0.10 (NS)
16	−0.42	0.29	0.09 (NS)
23	−1.13	0.04	0.02*
30	−1.88	−0.42	0.006**

VSS: Vancouver scar scale.
NS: not significant.
**Significant at 5%.*
***Significant at 1%.*

Table 3.
Average change in the VSS score of scars treated with silver sulfadiazine, vitamin A, and lidocaine (cream A) and with a cream without active ingredients (cream B) in patients with breast implants after 3, 6, 9, 16, 23, and 30 days from the onset of the topical treatment.

Days	Average change in the VSS score as from treatment onset (face and neck lift)		P
	Cream A	Cream B	
3	0.50	1.50	0.17 (NS)
6	0.13	1.50	0. 048*
9	−0.13	2.00	0.029*
16	−0.50	1.88	0.029*
23	−0.86	1.75	0.020*
30	−1.88	1.88	0.007**

VSS: Vancouver scar scale.
NS: not significant.
**Significant at 5%.*
***Significant at 1%.*

Table 4.
Average change in the VSS score of scars treated with silver sulfadiazine, vitamin A, and lidocaine (cream A) and with a cream without active ingredients (cream B) in patients with face lift after 3, 6, 9, 16, 23, and 30 days from the onset of the topical treatment.

those treated with cream B. On day 23, scars treated with cream A had decreased by 0.86 points average, while those treated with cream B had increased by 1.75 points average. On day 30, the average score decrease of scars treated with cream A was 1.88 points, while the score of scars treated with cream B increased by 1.88 average points (**Table 4**). **Figure 2** displays the changes in the VSS scores for each patient with breast implants on 23 and 30 days, compared to the initial control. In a majority of patients, we see a favorable effect with the cream A treatment compared to cream B, except for three cases (patients No. 16, 28, and 30). **Figure 3** illustrates the changes in the VSS scores for each patient with face and neck lifts on days 6, 9, 16, 23, and 30 with respect to the initial appointment. In most cases, cream A shows a more favorable effect in comparison with cream B. Regardless of whether cream A or B had been used, in general, the changes observed in the VSS, either increase or decrease, were homogeneous in the three variables that make up this scale: pigmentation, vascularity, and thickness of the scar. **Figures 4–6** illustrate the different results obtained when applying each cream.

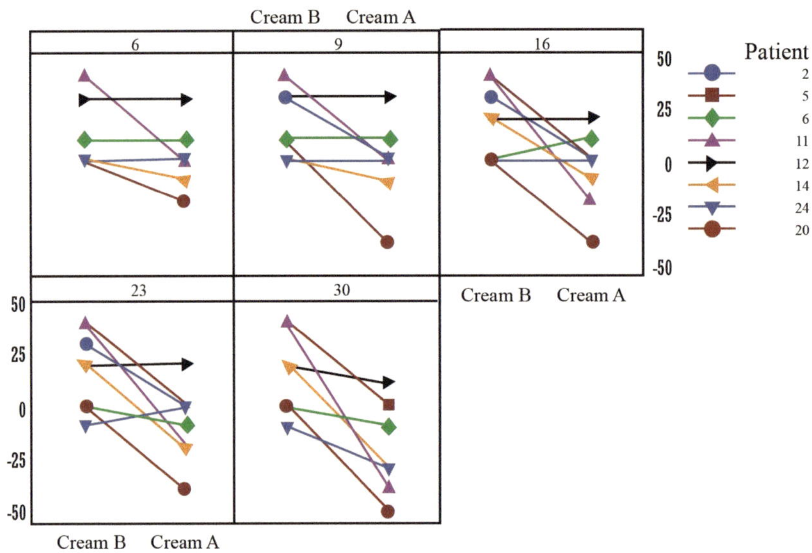

Figure 2.
Changes in VSS scores for each patient with breast implants after 23 and 30 days from treatment onset of treatment. VSS: Vancouver scar scale.

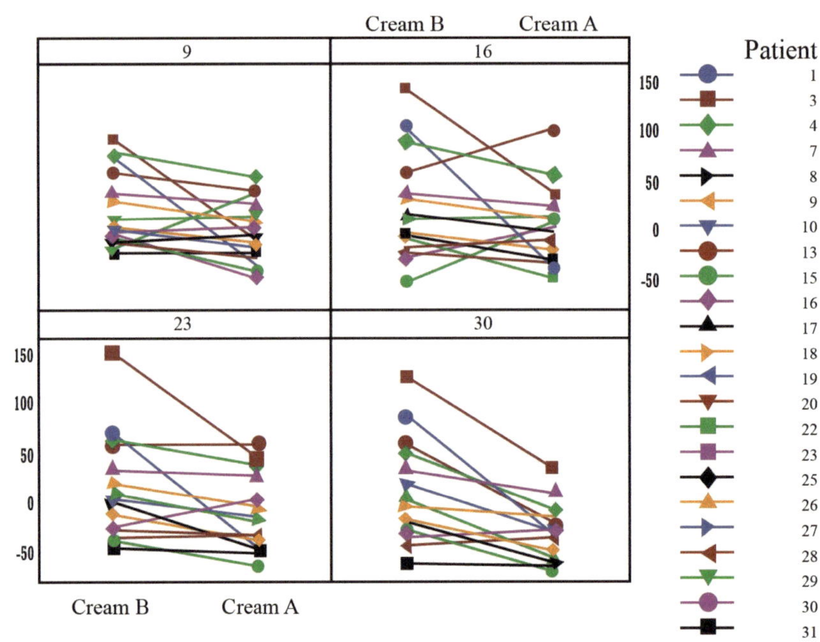

Figure 3.
Changes in VSS scores for each patient with cervical-facial stretch and after 6, 9, 16, 23, and 30 days from treatment onset. VSS: Vancouver scar scale.

2.3 Patient and observer objective assessment scale

This scale allowed us to evaluate numerically, based on the patient's own answers, scar characteristics related to pain, itching, color, stiffness, and thickness. The treating physician recorded the data reported for each variable and for each scar during the corresponding appointments. Although the score may vary between 0 and 60, the average of the initial scores was 16 and the maximum value observed throughout the study was 25. We carried out the analysis taking into account the

DOI: http://dx.doi.org/10.5772/intechopen.84127

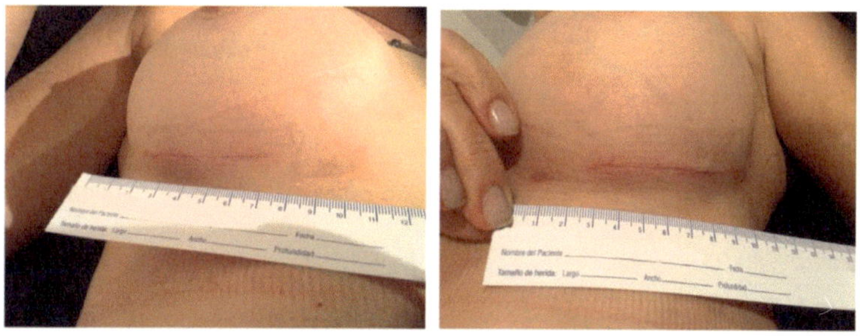

Figure 4.
Same patient's evolution with cream A (left) versus cream B (right) following a breast implant intervention (submammary incision).

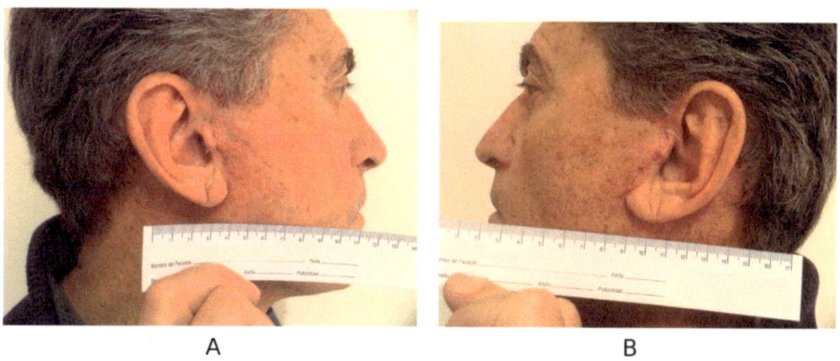

Figure 5.
Same patient's evolution with cream A (left) versus cream B (right) following a face lift intervention.

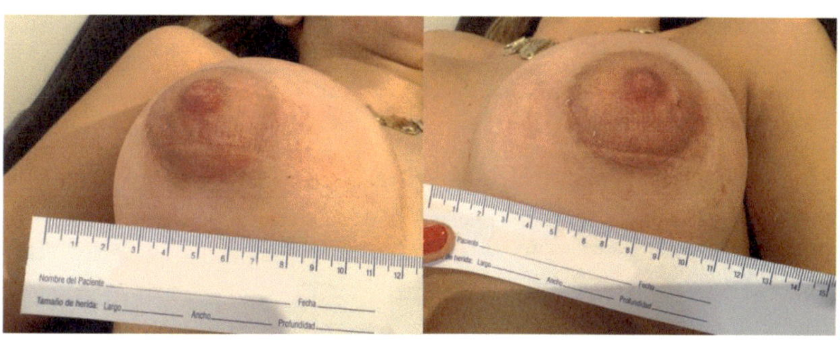

Figure 6.
Same patient's evolution with cream A (left) versus cream B (right) following a breast implant intervention (periareolar incision).

percentage change in the score of the scale with respect to that of the beginning of the treatment (day 0). We evaluated the results separately for each group of patients, depending on the type of surgery performed, and we considered the results obtained on days 3, 6, 9, 16, 23, and 30 of the postoperative period.

In the group of patients with breast implants, the percentage change of the score of the POSAS did not differ significantly between the treatments on days 3 and 6, but in the remaining appointments, we found a statistically significant difference ($P < 0.05$) in favor of cream A. The percentage decrease in the score was significantly higher in those scars treated with cream A than in those treated with cream B. On day 23, the score of scars treated with cream A decreased by

Days	Average change in the POSAS score as from treatment onset (face and neck lift)		P
	Cream A	Cream B	
3	2.5	8.5	1.0 (NS)
6	1.7	7.8	0.129 (NS)
9	−6.2	7.1	0.026*
16	−9.9	6.6	0.037*
23	−21.8	−1.3	0.005**
30	−37.7	−7.3	0.0007**

POSAS: patient and observer scar assessment scale.
NS: not significant.
**Significant at 5%.*
***Significant at 1%.*

Table 5.
Average POSAS score change rate for scars with silver sulfadiazine, vitamin A, and lidocaine (cream A) and with a cream without active ingredients (cream B) in patients with breast implants after 3, 6, 9, 16, 23, and 30 days from the onset of the topical treatment.

Days	Average change in the POSAS score as from treatment onset (breast implant)		P
	Cream A	Cream B	
3	22.1	18.2	0.66 (NS)
6	18.2	20.2	0.40 (NS)
9	19.0	26.3	0.26 (NS)
16	18.0	23.9	0.36 (NS)
23	−1.4	32.7	0.07 (NS)
30	−14.4	26.6	0.021*

POSAS: patient and observer scar assessment scale.
NS: not significant.
**Significant at 5%.*

Table 6.
Average POSAS score change rate for scars with silver sulfadiazine, vitamin A, and lidocaine (cream A) and with a cream without active ingredients (cream B) in patients with face lift after 3, 6, 9, 16, 23, and 30 days from the onset of the topical treatment.

21.8 points average, while that of the scars treated with cream B did so by 1.3 points average. On day 30, the average score decrease was of 37.7 points in scars treated with cream A while, in those treated with cream B, the decrease was 7.3 points average (**Table 5**).

In the group of patients with face and neck lifts, the percentage change in the POSAS score did not differ significantly between the treatments on days 3, 6, 9, 16, and 23. On day 30, however, we detected a statistically significant difference ($P = 0.021$) in favor of cream A. The percentage decrease was significantly higher in cases treated with cream A versus those treated with cream B. On day 30, the score of scars treated with cream A decreased, on average, by 14.4%, while that of the scars treated with cream B increased, on average, by 26.6% (**Table 6**). **Figure 7** presents the percentage changes of the POSAS scores for each patient with breast implants on days 9, 16, 23, and 30 with respect to the initial appointment,

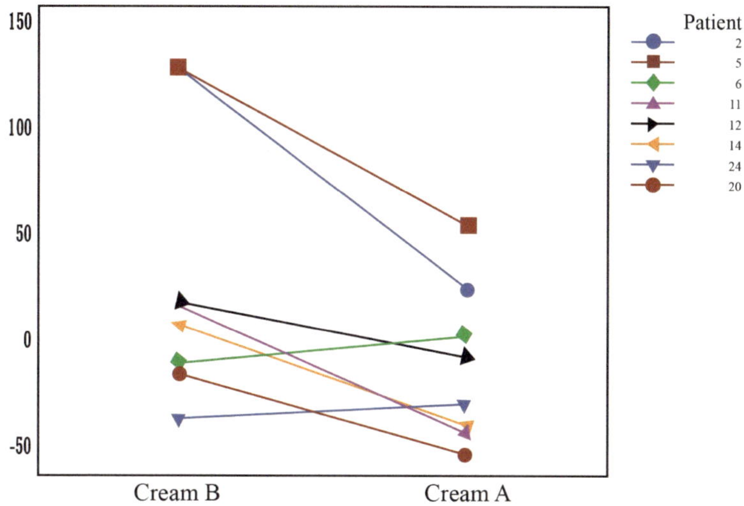

Figure 7.
Percentage POSAS score changes for each patient with breast implants after 9, 16, 23, and 30 days from the beginning of treatment. POSAS: patient and observer objective evaluation scale.

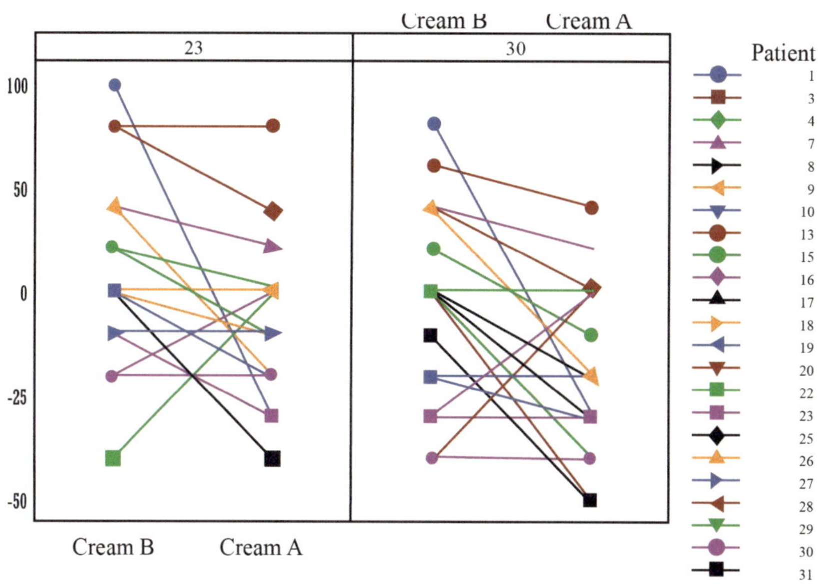

Figure 8.
POSAS score changes for each patient with face lift after 30 days from treatment onset. POSAS: patient and observer objective evaluation scale.

differentiated according to the treatment applied. In most patients, we see that the treatment with cream A resulted in a more favorable effect than that obtained with cream B, except for two cases (patient No. 15, days 9 and 16; and patient No. 13, day 16). **Figure 8** shows the percentage changes of the POSAS scores for each patient with face and neck lift between the onset of the treatment and day 30 and organizes the results based on the cream employed. In most cases, a better outcome was reached with cream A than with cream B. Irrespective of the cream applied, in general, the changes observed, either increase or decrease, reflected homogeneous changes in the variables that constitute this scale.

The results showed an improvement of all the evaluated variables when we used the cream with silver sulfadiazine, vitamin A, and lidocaine as treatment [6]. In all the scars treated in this way, we observed a greater percentage decrease of the surface area as compared with those treated with the cream without active principles. In addition, the scars treated with silver sulfadiazine, vitamin A, and lidocaine obtained a lower POSAS score, associated with a better scar quality. Such decrease in the POSAS score throughout the treatment is indicative not only of a more positive perception by the patient of the healing process but also of improvement of all the parameters evaluated: pain, itching, color, stiffness, thickness, and irregular scarring [7]. Therefore, our results indicate that performing a topical treatment with a cream containing silver sulfadiazine, vitamin A, and lidocaine from the beginning of treatment decreases wound size faster, improves the quality of the scar and the overall perception of the patients. In other words, such a treatment of postcosmetic surgery scars yields better esthetic and functional outcomes [8].

3. Combining skin substitutes for dermal reconstruction

The other treatment we are concerned with involves using different dermal substitutes in reconstructive surgery. Soft tissue impairment after an accident requires fast radical treatment and often multiple surgical procedures related to necrotic and poorly perfused tissue. Traditionally, dermal reconstruction meant harvesting grafts and flaps, which left major sequelae in donor sites. However, modern understanding of the composition of the skin has enabled researchers to develop numerous cutaneous substitutes which allow for the reconstruction of the dermis by providing a scaffold that promotes new tissue growth, thus compensating for the functional and physiological impairments caused by damaged tissue. Moreover, they offer the attractive possibility of employing grafts to treat large burns.

Skin substitutes are biomatrices that may be used to replace the damaged epidermis or dermis (or both) partially or totally, transitory or definitively. Although they can be classified in different ways [9], they fall broadly into two groups, either decellularized dermis derived from human or animal sources or artificially constructed scaffolds comprised of highly purified biomaterials or synthetic polymers. Many of these substitutes act by guiding the patient's own cells to form a neodermis, both reducing pain and improving healing by avoiding excessive scarring [10]. They allow practitioners to create a controlled environment appropriate for physiology and cellular function, as well as to identify and properly manipulate the cells so that parenchyma, stroma, and vascular components are generated, and to produce materials malleable by the cells.

One such cutaneous substitute is Integra®, which consists of a matrix of purified collagen from bovine tendon cross-linked with glycosaminoglycan obtained from shark cartilage and a silicone layer that functions as a temporary epidermis. It is a bilayer membrane system, consisting of an inner dermal substitute layer and a temporary outer epidermal substance layer. The inner layer is composed of a three-dimensional matrix of cross-linked bovine tendon collagen plus a glycosaminoglycan, and the outer layer is made of silicone. Integra® was introduced by Burke and Yannas in the early 1980s. The aim of their research was to find a substitute for the skin of patients with massive burns [11]. Nowadays, Integra® is a fundamental part of the "reconstructive ladder" and is utilized for treating skin loss resulting from burns, trauma and oncologic and pressure sore surgery [12]. After application of Integra®, the patient's native fibroblasts, macrophages, and lymphocytes infiltrate and new capillary growth occurs into the matrix of the inner layer. The inner layer becomes degraded and an endogenous collagen matrix is deposited by the patient's own fibroblasts, forming a neodermis. Once engraftment is complete, 2–3 weeks after application, the outer silicone layer needs to be removed and an epidermal autograft must be placed over the neodermis. One of the advantages of this process is that successful neodermis formation requires only a thin skin graft which provides epidermal coverage which also prevents infections. Furthermore, as no donor site is created, it eliminates the risk of donor site wound complications.

Another skin substitute is cadaver skin or homograft, which was included in protocols for the first time in the year 1981 in Philadelphia, United States. By virtue of the processing of cadaver skin through a skin bank, a suitable substitute is obtained and distributed to potential receptors [13]. Depending on the way in which they are processed, these "acellular dermal homografts" (as Takami describes them [14]) can be used transiently or permanently. To reduce the probability of graft rejection, cadaveric grafts undergo a cell-removal process and the resulting acellular tissue is irradiated with gamma rays, which destroy the immunogenic potential of the tissue. Employing cadaver skin to treat severe trauma of lower limbs with skin impairment has a number of advantages. To begin with, this treatment produces a biological closure after escharectomy. Furthermore, it helps reduce the loss of fluids, proteins, and electrolytes, as well as the pain experienced by the patient. Apart from this, it prevents the desiccation of the wound bed, since it functions as a biological cover for complex wounds, ultimately improving the preparation of the wound bed before definite reconstruction [15]. Finally, the addition of artificial skin over the vascularized homologous dermis creates a dermal structure of greater thickness and elasticity.

Another recent development which is of great importance for reconstructive surgery is vacuum therapy (VAC), which improves wound healing by means of two main mechanisms. In the first place, it acts on the interstitial level eliminating edema, inflammatory mediators, and bacteria. It thus combats the vicious cycle of increased interstitial edema and pressure, cell death, and necrosis which is begotten by the inflammatory response triggered after a lesion. In addition, this treatment promotes mitogenesis and granulation tissue formation [16]. VAC is relevant to our research since, as Morykwas explains, it can be used to help incorporate Integra® and skin grafts as permanent replacements. Using a vacuum system after the escharectomy and the homograft placement and 1 week after positioning the artificial skin and the ultrathin autograft favors the arrest of these two substitutes. Moreover, negative pressure wound therapy can help augment the healing process and prepare the wound for definitive closure. A review published in Cochrane in 2007 [21] reported that, after 6 months of treatment, a 71% success rate had been observed in wounds treated with both artificial skin and negative pressure through

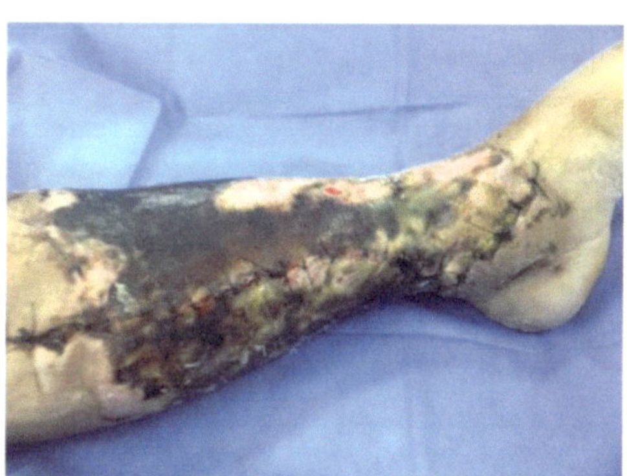

Figure 9.
Full-thickness trauma in lower limbs.

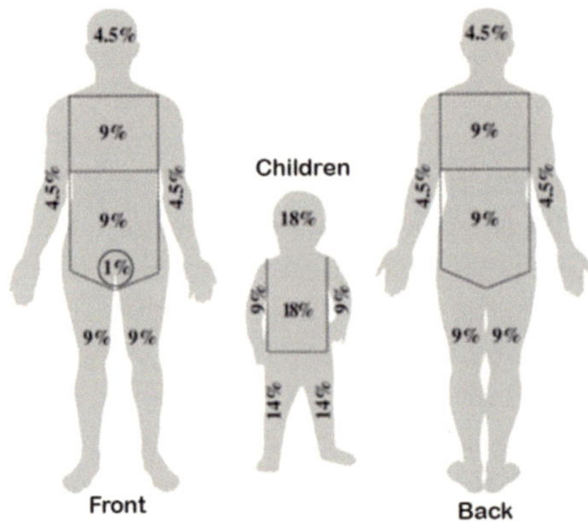

Figure 10.
Pulaski and Tennison's Rules of Nines.

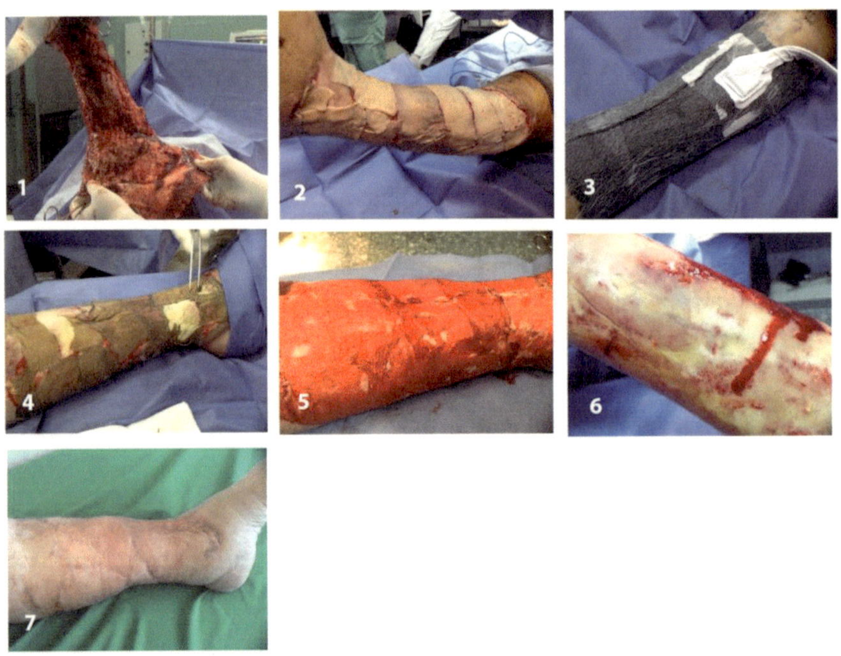

Figure 11.
(1) Escharectomy, (2) cadaver skin, (3) vacuum system, (4) epidermolysis, (5) neovascularized homodermis, and (6) artificial skin over vascularized homodermis—final result with autograft.

a vacuum system, whereas the success rate of wounds treated solely with negative pressure had been, at 37%, significantly lower. In terms of wound healing, even better results were obtained when Integra® was used as a dermal substitute [22].

As a consequence of the benefits we have mentioned, dermal substitutes have now been extended to treat other pathologies. Furthermore, the use of cutaneous substitutes added to the vacuum therapy has been incorporated into the "Modified Ladder of Reconstruction" [17]. However, the usefulness of treating large wounds with deep skin impairment with both cadaver skin and artificial skins has not been, to date, exhaustively studied. Therefore, we wish to contribute to this line of research by reporting the successful esthetic and functional results we have obtained when treating extensive skin lesions with both substitutes. Our study involved the follow-up of the wound healing of four patients (N:4) who had suffered high impact trauma in their lower

Grade	Definition
Grade 1	Any deviation from the normal postoperative course without the need for pharmacological treatment or surgical, endoscopic, and radiological interventions Allowed therapeutic regiments are: drugs and antiemetics, antipyretics, analgetics, diuretics, electrolytes, and physiotherapy. This grade also includes wound infections opened at the bedside
Grade 2	Requiring pharmacological treatment with drugs other than such allowed for grade 1 complications. Blood transfusions and total parenteral nutrition are also included
Grade 3	Requiring surgical, endoscopic, or radiological intervention
Grade 3a	Intervention not under general anesthesia
Grade 3b	Intervention under general anesthesia
Grade 4	Life-threatening complications including brain hemorrhage, ischemic stroke, subarachnoid bleeding, and central nervous system complications (but excluding transient ischemic attacks) requiring intermediate care or intensive care unit management
Grade 4a	Single organ dysfunction (including dialysis)
Grade 4b	Multiorgan dysfunction
Grade 5	Death of a patient
Suffix "d"	If the patient suffers from a complication at the time of discharge, the suffix "d" (for "disability") is added to the respective grade of complication. This label indicates the need for a follow-up to fully evaluate the complication

Table 7.
Dindo classification of surgical complications.

limbs (**Figure 9**) and who were treated at Hospital Alemán in the city of Buenos Aires. All of them were females with ages ranging from 19 to 73 years (median: 32 years). All of their lesions belonged to Group 4 of Benaim's severity classification and ranked as full-thickness burns in Benaim's depth classification [18]. The affected body surface was calculated based on the rule of nines described by Pulaski and Tennison in 1949 [19] (**Figure 10**) with the following results: 8% in the 19-year-old patient, 24% in the 22-year-old, 28% in the 43-year-old, and 8% in the 73-year-old (**Table 4**).

In all cases, escharectomy was performed on fascia within the first 48 h of the accident. Immediately afterward, the wounds were covered with cadaver skin from the tissue bank. Over the next 5–9 days, epidermolysis was observed (i.e., spontaneous removal of the epidermis), as well as vascularization and arrest of the homologous dermis on the receptor bed. In the second stage, the artificial skin was placed on the built-in vascularized homologous dermis. Once the artificial skin had been placed, we waited for 21 days before removing the silicone layer and completing the third and last surgical stage with the placement of a 1/4-thick autograft, obtained with an electric dermatome, over the heterologous vascularized neodermis. **Figure 11** illustrates the procedure we followed and the results we obtained.

We used a grid of manual design to evaluate the arrest of the cadaver and artificial skin (expressed in percentages). The arrest of the cadaver skin was of 95% and the placement of the heterologous matrix with an ultrathin autograft was of 94%. The average hospital time was 46 days. No major complications were present, but only minimal difficulties belonging to grades 3b, 4, and 5 of the Dindo and Clavien table [20] (**Table 7**). After a year of follow-up, we observed that favorable functional results had been obtained in highly complex articular areas such as ankles or knees due to the contribution of homologous and heterologous matrixes that provided adequate scaffolding. With respect to the esthetic results, no depression of the covered surfaces was observed with respect to the adjacent normal dermal tissue. Furthermore, there was no evidence of pathological scarring (such as keloids or hypertrophic scars).

4. Conclusions

The goal of any healing process is not only that the scar does not bring about functional disruptions, but also that it is as inconspicuous as possible. Patients of both cosmetic and reconstructive surgery expect scars that do not stand out from the normal surrounding skin, yet there is no consensus among medical practitioners as to which healing methods can achieve both functional and esthetic goals most effectively. In this chapter, we have accounted for two studies carried out at Hospital Alemán in the city of Buenos Aires, the promising results of which may help practitioners arrive at a standard for treating scars resulting from cosmetic and reconstructive surgery.

Regarding postcosmetic surgery scars, we have tested the progress of the scars of 32 patients, each having two postsurgical scars that were treated with two different creams. The results of our research show that performing a topical treatment with a cream that contains silver sulfadiazine, vitamin A, and lidocaine from the onset of the treatment decreases the size of the wound more quickly, improves the quality of the scar and the patient's perception of it. These findings contrast with the less positive outcome of the scars treated with a moisturizing cream without active ingredients [23]. Thus, we conclude that using creams with active ingredients should be promoted as a common practice.

In turn, in our study related to reconstructive surgery, we followed the progress of four patients whose massive skin loss was treated with a combination of artificial and cadaveric dermal substitutes. Using modern biotechnology to reconstruct damaged structures and to provide a new extracellular matrix constitutes the greatest breakthrough in reconstructive surgery of recent times. The development of homografts and artificial skin has allowed professionals to accelerate healing by covering wounds transitorily or permanently. At the same time, they work as a barrier against infections, help maintain the hydroelectrolytic balance [24], and improve esthetic and functional results. As we explained in the previous section, the quality of the scar and the properties of the neodermis depend on the use of an appropriate extracellular matrix [25].

As part of our research, we assessed the progress of the four patients' scars, focusing on such characteristics as color, thickness, volume, and pain, as well as on the restoration of function at affected sites. We noted positive outcomes in all evaluated parameters, which points at the advantages entailed in implementing this technique. Moreover, the number of hypertrophic scars was lower than the average. Our method fulfilled the ultimate goal of tissue engineering, namely, to restore damaged or lost tissue in traumatic wounds that result in a functional barrier, providing, at the same time, for rapid closure to prevent dehydration and bacterial infection. As attested by our results, the advantages of combining both dermal substitutes include better functional and esthetic outcomes, pain relief, and enhancement of the overall quality of the scar.

All in all, the results of both studies are indicative of the direction that modern scar treatment can take in order to achieve the desired goals in both cosmetic and reconstructive surgery. In the case of the former, achieving an esthetically pleasing scar has long been recognized as a fundamental requirement of a successful intervention. Here, the most optimal results can be achieved if wound treatment and care are initiated early. However, the esthetic factor should not be limited to this type of procedures. Our work on reconstructive surgery centers around the concept that such surgery should not only merely aim at "rebuilding" but also at obtaining the best functional and esthetic outcome with the least possible number of interventions. Recent advances in biotechnology offer us effective skin substitutes, which can be combined so as to achieve a better evolution of the wounds. [26] Such improved esthetic and functional results in posttraumatic reconstructive surgery ensure an ad integrum recovery of the affected areas, which, ultimately, enhances the quality of patients' lives.

DOI: http://dx.doi.org/10.5772/intechopen.84127

Author details

Gustavo E. Prezzavento
Hospital Alemán, Buenos Aires, Argentina

*Address all correspondence to: prezzavento.gustavo@gmail.com

References

[1] Glat PM, Longaker MT. Wound healing. In: Aston SJ, Beasley RW, Thorne CH, editors. Grabb and Smith's Plastic Surgery. 5th ed. Philadelphia: Lippencott; 1997. pp. 3-12

[2] Mordon S, Trelles MA. Advantages of laser assisted scar healing (LASH). Cirugía Plástica Ibero-Latinoamericana. 2011;**37**(4):387-392

[3] Andrades P, Benitez S, Prado A. Guidelines for the treatment of kelloids and hipertrophic scars. Revista Chilena de Cirugía, Santiago de Chile, Chile. 2006;**58**(2):78-88

[4] Sullivan T, Smith J, Kermode J, et al. Rating the burn scar. The Journal of Burn Care & Rehabilitation. 1990;**11**:256-260

[5] Draaijers L, Tempelman F, Botman Y, et al. The patient and observer scar assessment scale: A reliable and feasible tool for scar evaluation. Plastic and Reconstructive Surgery. 2004;**113**:1960-1965

[6] Hunt TK. Vitamin A and wound healing. Journal of the American Academy of Dermatology. 1986;**15**:817-821

[7] Robson MC. Wound infection. A failure of wound healing caused by an imbalance of bacteria. The Surgical Clinics of North America. 1997;**77**:637-650

[8] Parsons D, Bowler PG, Myles V, et al. Silver antimicrobial dressings in wound management: A comparison of antibacterial, physical, and chemical characteristics. Wounds. 2005;**17**:222-232

[9] Leclerc T, Thepenier PJ, Bey E, Peltzer J, Trouillas M, Duhamel P, et al. Cell therapy of burns. Cell Proliferation. 2011;**44**:48-54

[10] Lee KH. Tissue-engineered human living skin substitutes: Development and clinical application. Yonsei Medical Journal. 2000;**41**:774-779

[11] Andreadis ST, Hamoen KE, Yarmush ML, Morgan JR. Keratinocyte growth factor induces hyperproliferation and delays differentiation in a skin equivalent model system. The FASEB Journal. 2001;**15**:898-906

[12] Leventhal D, Furr M, Reiter D. Treatment of keloids and hypertrophic scars. Archives of Facial Plastic Surgery. 2006;**8**:362-368

[13] May SR, De Clement FA. Skin banking methodology; an eva- luation of package format, cooling and warming rates, storage,efficiency. Cryobiology. 1970;**17**:33

[14] Takami Y, Matsuda T, et al. Dispas/detergent treated dermal matrix as a dermal substitute. Burns. 1996;**22**:182-290

[15] Moerman E et al. The temporary use of allograft for complicated wounds in plastic surgery. Burns. 2002;**28**(Suppl. 1): S13-S15

[16] Sanger C, Molnar JA, Newman CE, et al. Poster 37: Immediate skin grafting of an engineered dermal substitute. Plastic and Reconstructive Surgery. 2005;**116**(35). American Society of Plastic Surgery, Plastic Surgery 2005. Chicago, IL. 24-28 Sept

[17] Janis JE, Kwon R, et al. The new reconstructive ladder: Modifications to the traditional model. Plastic and Reconstructive Surgery. 2011;**127**(Suppl. 1)

[18] Benaim F. Enfoque global del tratamiento de las quemaduras. In: Coiffman F editors. Cirugía plástica recosntructiva y estética. Barcelona, España: Editorial Masson-Salvat; 1994. pp. 443-4961

[19] Knaysi GA, Crikelair GF, et al. The rule of nine's; its history and accuracy. Plastic and Reconstructive Surgery. 1968;**41**:560-563

[20] Dindo D, Demartines N, et al. Classification of surgical complications: A new proposal with evaluation in a cohort of 6336 patients and results of a survey. Annals of Surgery. 2004;**240**:205-213

[21] Jones GE, Nelson EA. Skin grafting for venous leg ulcers (review). The Cochrane collaboration; 2007

[22] Pham C, Greenwood J, et al. Bioengineered skin substitutes for the management of burns: A systematic review. Burns. 2007;**33**:946-957

[23] Prezzavento GE, Racca L, Bottai H. Scarring: An evaluation of two topical treatments commonly used in post-aesthetic surgery scar. Cir. plást. iberolatinoam. 2017;**43**(3):255-263

[24] Eisenbud D, Huang NF, et al. Skin substitutes and wound healing: Current status and challenges. Wounds. 2004;**16**(1):2-17

[25] Kagan RJ, Robb EC, Plessinger RT. Human skin banking. Clinics in Laboratory Medicine. 2005;**25**:587-605

[26] Prezzavento G. Skin substitutes. Can these be combined? (review). Journal of Embryology & Stem Cell Research. 2018;**2**(1):000104